AF820981

Renal Physiology and Biochemistry

International Journal of Experimental Renal Physiology, Pathophysiology, Biochemistry and Pharmacology

Founded 1978 by G.M. Berlyne and S. Thomas

KARGER

Printed in Switzerland
on acid-free paper by
Reinhardt Druck, Basel

Appears bimonthly:
1 volume per year (6 issues)

Renal Physiology and Biochemistry

Submission: Only original papers written in English are considered and should be sent to:

S. Karger AG
Editorial Dept. 'Renal Physiology and Biochemistry'
P.O. Box
CH-4009 Basel (Switzerland)

Manuscripts should be submitted in quadruplicate (with four sets of illustrations of which one is an original), typewritten double-spaced on one side of the paper, with a wide margin.
Rapid communications: Manuscripts intended for rapid communication must present new findings of sufficient importance to justify their accelerated appearance. Double-spaced manuscripts cannot exceed 5½ pages, including figures, tables and references; longer manuscripts will be returned. The manuscripts will be seen by two referees and one of the editors, and the decision, accepted, returned for minor revisions or rejected, will be made within 1 month. The manuscripts are published within 4 months following acceptance. Proofs are checked by the Editor and not sent to the authors.

Conditions: All manuscripts are subject to editorial review. Manuscripts are received with the explicit understanding that they are not under simultaneous consideration by any other publication. Submission of an article for publication implies the transfer of the copyright from the author to the publisher upon acceptance. Accepted papers become the permanent property of 'Renal Physiology and Biochemistry' and may not be reproduced by any means, in whole or in part, without the written consent of the publisher. It is the author's responsibility to obtain permission to reproduce illustrations, tables, etc. from other publications.

Arrangement
Title page: The first page of each paper should indicate the title (main title underlined), the authors' names, and the institute where the work was conducted. A short title for use as running head as well as the full address of the author to whom correspondence should be sent are also required.
Full address: The exact postal address complete with postal code must be given at the bottom of the title page. Please also supply Phone and Fax numbers.
Key words: For indexing purposes, a list of 3–10 key words in English is essential.
Abstract: Each paper needs an abstract of up to 10 lines.
Small type: Paragraphs which can or must be set in smaller type (case histories, test methods, etc.) should be indicated with a 'p' (petit) in the margin on the left-hand side.
Footnotes: Avoid footnotes. When essential, they are numbered consecutively and typed at the foot of the appropriate page.
Tables and illustrations: Tables and illustrations (both numbered in Arabic numerals) should be prepared on separate sheets. Tables require a heading and figures a legend, also prepared on a separate sheet. For the reproduction of illustrations, only good drawings and original photographs can be accepted; negatives or photocopies cannot be used. When possible, group several illustrations on one block for reproduction (max. size 144 × 196 mm) or provide crop marks. On the back of each illustration, indicate its number, the author's name, and 'top'. Color illustrations are reproduced at the author's expense.
References: In the text identify references by Arabic numerals [in square brackets]. Material submitted for publication but not yet accepted should be noted as 'unpublished data' and not be included in the reference list. The list of references should include only those publications which are cited in the text. Do not alphabetize; number references in the order in which they are first mentioned in the text. The surnames of the authors followed by initials should be given. There should be no punctuation other than a comma to separate the authors. Cite all authors, 'et al' is not sufficient. Abbreviate journal names according to the Index Medicus system. (Also see International Committee of Medical Journal Editors: Uniform requirements for manuscripts submitted to biomedical journals. Br Med J 1988;296:401–405.)
Examples
(a) Papers published in periodicals: Kauffman HF, van der Heide S, Beaumont F, Blok H, de Vries K: Class-specific antibody determination against *Aspergillus fumigatus* by means of the enzyme-linked immunosorbent assay. III. Comparative study: IgG, IgA, IgM ELISA titers, precipitating antibodies and IgE binding after fractionation of the antigen. Int Arch Allergy Appl Immunol 1986;80:300–306.
(b) Monographs: Matthews DE, Farewell VT: Using and Understanding Medical Statistics. Basel, Karger, 1985.
(c) Edited books: Hardy WD Jr, Essex M: FeLV-induced feline acquired immune deficiency syndrome: A model for human AIDS; in Klein E (ed): Acquired Immunodeficiency Syndrome. Prog Allergy. Basel, Karger, 1986, vol 37, pp 353–376.
Further details: Authors may consult our leaflet 'Rules for the Preparation of Manuscripts', available on request from the Publisher, S. Karger AG, P.O. Box, CH-4009 Basel (Switzerland).

Page charges: A page charge of SFr. 115.– / US $ 75.00 per printed page will be levied (1 printed page is equal to approximately 2 manuscript pages including tables, illustrations and references).

Galley proofs: Unless indicated otherwise, galley proofs are sent to the first-named author and should be returned with the least possible delay. Alterations made in galley proofs, other than the correction of printer's errors, are charged to the author. No page proofs are supplied.

Reprints: Order forms and a price list are sent with the galley proofs. Orders submitted after the issue is printed are subject to considerably higher prices. Allow five weeks from date of publication for delivery of reprints.

KARGER

General Information

Renal Physiology and Biochemistry

Publication data: 'Renal Physiology and Biochemistry' is published 6 times annually. Volume 16 with 6 issues appears in 1993.
Subscription rates: Subscriptions run for a full calendar year. Prices are given per volume.
Personal subscription:
Subscription + postage and handling
SFr. 278.60 + SFr. 16.80 Europe
SFr. 278.60 + SFr. 25.20 Overseas
US$ 186.20 + US$ 16.80
(Must be in the name of, billed to, and paid by an individual. Order must be marked 'personal subscription'.)
Institutional subscription:
Subscription + postage and handling
SFr. 398.– + SFr. 24.– Europe
SFr. 398.– + SFr. 36.– Overseas
US$ 266.00 + US$ 24.00
Airmail postage: SFr. 36.–, US$ 30.00. (Extra per volume.)
Microform edition: SFr. 199.–, US$ 133.00. (Available exclusively to subscribers of the paper edition.)
Advertising: Correspondence and rate requests should be addressed to the Publisher.

Subscription orders: Orders can be placed at agencies, bookstores, directly with the Publisher S. Karger AG, P.O. Box, CH – 4009 Basel (Switzerland)
or with any of the following distributors:
Deutschland: S. Karger GmbH
Lörracher Strasse 16A, Postfach
D-W-7800 Freiburg
France: Librairie Luginbühl
36, bd de Latour-Maubourg
F-75007 Paris
Great Britain, Ireland: S. Karger Publishers
11 Ravenscroft Road
Beckenham, Kent BR3 4TP
USA: S. Karger Publishers, Inc.
26 West Avon Road, P.O. Box 529
Farmington, CT 06085
India, Bangladesh, Sri Lanka:
S. Karger India Subscription Agency
B – 5/132 Safdarjung Enclave
New Delhi-110029
Japan: Katakura Libri, Inc.
36-9 Hongo 3-chome, Bunkyo-ku
Tokyo 113
Change of address: Both old and new address should be sent to the subscription source.
Single issues and back volumes: Information can be obtained through the Publisher.

Bibliographic indices: This journal is regularly listed in bibliographic services, including *Current Contents®*.
Book Reviews: Books are accepted for review by special agreement.

Guidelines for Disk Submission

Karger Publishers welcomes the submission of manuscripts on disk.

Please observe the 'Instructions to authors' as well as the following guidelines:

Technical Data

The preferred **storage medium** is a 3.5- or 5.25-inch disk in MS-DOS format. Macintosh is also acceptable.

The preferred **word processing package** is Microsoft Word. Other commonly used PC text programs are also accepted, as well as ASCII formats.

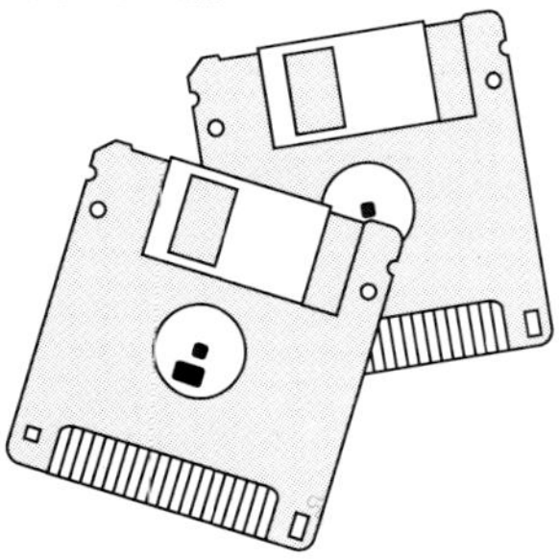

Handling

All manuscripts accepted for Karger publications are subject to copyediting. It is therefore essential that you send us a **double-spaced printout** of your manuscript which exactly matches the disk.

Any subsequent revised versions should be clearly marked as such, both on the disk and on the manuscript.

The copyedited manuscript and the disk will be returned to you along with the galley proofs. Please be sure to **check the galleys against the manuscript** in which changes introduced by the copyeditor and/or questions will be marked.

Please **label** your disk with (a) the title of the journal for which it is submitted, (b) a short version of the paper title, (c) your name and (d) the software and hardware used.

Text Arrangement

Text and headings should be ranged left throughout, without word breaks. **Do not center, space, or use block letters** for text and headings (except for abbreviations). **Do not use indentations** to mark the beginning of a paragraph, but use one blank line between paragraphs.

Be sure to use the **same type style for headings of the same ranking** throughout the text.

When using **special characters** not available on a standard keyboard (including Greek characters), please do so by a readily identifiable code, and use the same code throughout the manuscript. Supply a **complete list of the codes used** at the beginning of the text.

Illustrations, tables and mathematical formulae will be handled conventionally.

KARGER

Cellular Basis of Renal Function

Guest Editors
Natale G. De Santo, Naples
Giovambattista Capasso, Naples

39 figures and 7 tables, 1993

KARGER

S. Karger
Medical and Scientific Publishers
Basel·Freiburg·Paris·London
New York·New Delhi·Bangkok
Singapore·Tokyo·Sydney

Drug Dosage
The authors and the publisher have exerted every effort to ensure that drug selection and dosage set forth in this text are in accord with current recommendations and practice at the time of publication. However, in view of ongoing research, changes in government regulations, and the constant flow of information relating to drug therapy and drug reactions, the reader is urged to check the package insert for each drug for any change in indications and dosage and for added warnings and precautions. This is particularly important when the recommended agent is a new and/or infrequently employed drug.

Printed in Switzerland on acid-free paper by
Buchdruckerei Friedrich Reinhardt AG, Basel
ISBN 3-8055-5770-1

Contents

Natale Gaspare De Santo
Giovambattista Capasso

Editorial

In the last few years our understanding of the kidney function has been mainly related to the elucidation of the fundamental mechanisms involved in cellular and molecular aspects of renal cell biology. This has been mainly dependent on the development of new techniques and new concepts in membrane and transport physiology. The introduction of in vivo and in vitro microperfusion, the application of special glass microelectrodes and fluorescent methods, the use of isolated single membranes, the development of the patch-clamp technique and the more recent attempt to identify, isolate, express and clone individual transport molecules by powerful methods of molecular biology have greatly stimulated and contributed to our comprehension of renal function.

However, such a large body of information has constrained the clinical investigator to face a major problem: to try and integrate the complex and vastly expanded knowledge of the cellular and molecular aspects of renal function into clinical medicine.

The current volume was prepared to pursue two goals: first, to clarify our understanding of renal function by studies that place this problem into the forefront of biology of epithelial cells in general; second, by taking a molecular approach to renal physiology, it was intended to give an instrument to all workers in this important area and bring recent advances to the attention of medical scientists.

We hope that the description of the fascinating world of renal cell organization will contribute to the clarification of some of the most relevant clinical aspects of kidney function in health and disease; in addition, it was our aim to introduce specific recent issues in cellular and molecular physiology in order to raise new questions on the fundamental problems of renal function.

Renal Physiol Biochem 1993;16:6–14

Detlev Drenckhahn
Thomas Jöns
Alice Kollert-Jöns
Rainer Koob
Doris Kraemer
Susanne Wagner

Institute of Anatomy,
Julius-Maximilian University,
Würzburg, FRG

Cytoskeleton and Epithelial Polarity

Key Words
Microtubules
Membrane cytoskeleton
Na^+, K^+–ATPase
Anion exchanger 1
Kidney
Urinary bladder
Enterocytes

Abstract
The membrane surface of polarized epithelial cells can be divided in apical and basolateral domains that differ in molecular composition and function. Components of the cytoskeleton are involved in critical steps of both generation and maintenance of cell polarity. Generation of polarity is controlled by microtubules that serve as uniformly aligned and polarized cytoplasmic guiding structures for the vectorial and selective transport of Golgi-derived carrier vesicles to the apical cell surface. Targeting of membrane proteins to the basolateral cell surface does not depend on microtubules but follows the constitutive bulk flow of membranes. Once inserted into the lipid bilayer several membrane proteins such as the kidney anion exchanger 1 (AE1) and the sodium pump become immobilized at specialized microdomains of the lateral cell surface. Evidence is provided that both membrane proteins are linked via ankyrin to the spectrin-based membrane cytoskeleton that underlies the basolateral membrane domain. Linkage of these and other integral membrane proteins to the cytoskeleton may not only place them to specialized sites of the plasma membrane but may also prevent these transporters from clustering and endocytosis, thus helping them to stay at the cell surface. In search of sequence motifs involved in binding of integral membrane proteins to components of the cytoskeleton we found that the binding interface of AE1 to protein 4.1 (an actin and spectrin cross-linking protein) consists of a cluster of five amino acid residues, namely IRRRY in AE1 and LEEDY on protein 4.1. This motif may play a more general role in cytoskeleton membrane linkages.

Detlev Drenckhahn
Institute of Anatomy
Julius-Maximilians-University
D-W-8700 Würzburg (FRG)

1011–6524/93/
0162–0006 $2.75/0

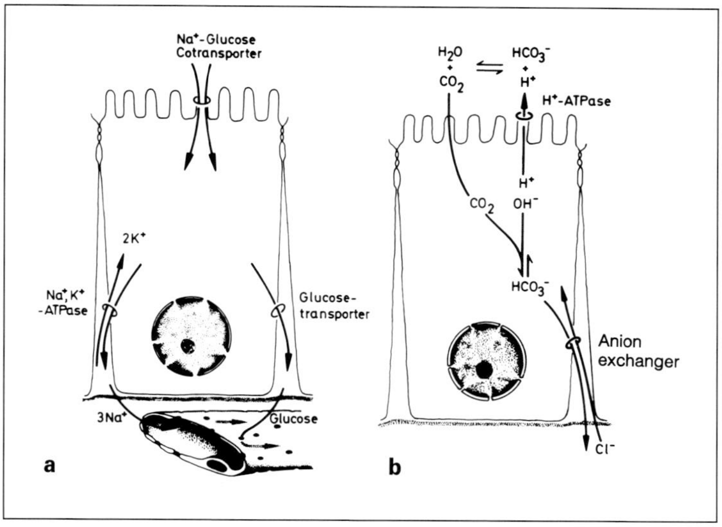

Fig. 1. Examples of molecular heterogeneity of the apical and basolateral plasma membrane in the intestinal epithelium (**a**) and type A intercalated cells of kidney collecting duct (**b**).

Introduction

Transporting epithelia, such as the epithelial lining of kidney tubules or the intestine, provide classical examples of polarized cell types that are capable of directing the transport of molecules and ions across the epithelial layer and of generating steep transepithelial electrochemical gradients. These functional properties of transporting epithelial cells depend to a large degree on the polarized compartmentalization of specific pumps, carriers, channels, and ectoenzymes to either the apical or basolateral membrane surface. The sodium pump (Na^+,K^+ATPase) and anion exchanger 1 (AE1) of kidney tubules are two examples of membrane proteins that are restricted to the basolateral domain of the plasma membrane [1–4]. The sodium pump is the major driving force for resorption of glucose and other solutes via sodium-coupled carriers which are confined to the apical cell surface. The basolateral AE1 of the kidney collecting duct and turtle urinary bladder allows resorption of $HC0_3^-$ ions that are left behind in the cytosol due to the activity of an apically located proton pump that translocates H^+ ions across the apical plasma membrane [5–7] (fig. 1). This striking asymmetric distribution of certain membrane proteins to either the apical or basolateral membrane domain raises the question of how this molecular polarity is generated and how it is maintained. Tight junctions (zonula occludens) which separate the apical and the basolateral membrane domains of polarized epithelial cells from each other are generally thought to act as a kind of fence within the lipid bilayer and thus to contribute to the maintenance of cell polarity by serving as a diffusion barrier for proteins and glycolipids between the apical and basolateral membrane domain [8, 9]. However, tight junctions cannot explain how membrane proteins are vectorially delivered from the Golgi apparatus to either the apical or basolateral cell surface. Moreover, thight junctions do obviously not play any role in restriction or placement of certain membrane proteins to specialized microdomains within the apical or basolateral cell surface. Examples of

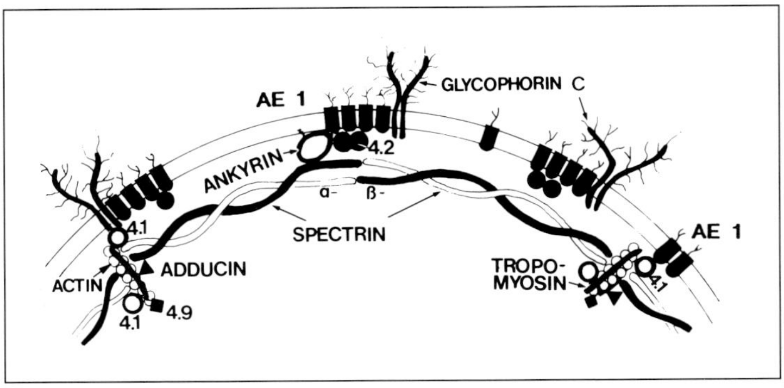

Fig. 2. Organization of the membrane cytoskeleton in erythrocytes.

such microdomains are pleated and folded portions of the basolateral cell surface of intercalated cells in the collecting duct. These folded areas are the main sites of renal AE1 which is absent from the plain areas of the plasma membrane.

One possible mechanism how particular membrane proteins could be localized and immobilized at specialized areas of the cell surface could be the linkage of these proteins to components of the membrane cytoskeleton. The membrane of erythrocytes provides an example of how an integral membrane protein, namely AE1 (also termed band 3), is connected via ankyrin and protein 4.1 to the fibrous meshwork comprised of spectrin, actin and several associated proteins [10, 11] (fig. 2). In this review the question of how components of the cytoskeleton may contribute to both generation and maintenance of cell polarity is addressed. The first part deals with the role of microtubules in the vectorial delivery of membrane proteins to the apical cell surface. The second part summarizes our current view on the function of components of the membrane cytoskeleton in restricting AE1 and the sodium pump to morphologically defined subdomains of the lateral cell surface.

Role of Microtubules in Epithelial Polarity

Several lines of evidence suggest that the Golgi apparatus and its associated transnetwork play an important role in the process of sorting membrane proteins into different populations of carrier vesicles that will be subsequently delivered and inserted into either the apical or the basolateral cell surface [12]. From experiments with microtubule (MT)-disrupting agents it has been concluded that MTs are involved in the generation of cell polarity by a still unknown mechanism.

By immunocytochemistry at the light- and electron-microscopic level we found in the intestinal epithelium and in other transporting epithelial cells that MTs display a preferential orientation parallel to the long axis of these columnar cells. This pattern of MTs differs profoundly from that in nonpolarized cell types where MTs emanate and fan out from the centrosome which is always located in vicinity of the nucleus. In polarized epithelial cells MTs are uniformly oriented towards a narrow space underneath the apical terminal web (termed subterminal space) that contains MT-organizing properties and controls polarized alignment of MTs in these cells [13]. Since the MT-organizing center is located underneath the apical cell surface epithelial microtubules probably contain the same polarity with the slowly growing end (minus end) located apically and the fast growing end basally (fig. 3). In other cell systems MTs have been shown to serve as tracks or guiding structures for the intracellular transport of organelles. The direction of transport depends on the type of MT motor protein associated with these carrier vesicles. Kinesin-like motor proteins have been shown in other cell types to carry vesicles to the plus end whereas dynein-like motors mediate transport to the minus end of MTs [14].

To obtain further insight into the role of MTs in cellular polarity targeting of three apical and one basolateral membrane protein was studied in the intestinal epithelium of rats and mice treated with the MT-depolymerizing drugs colchicine and vinblastine [15]. These experiments showed that depolymerization of MTs selectively interferes with polarized delivery of membrane proteins destined for the apical plasma membrane (isomaltase, aminopeptidase, alkaline phosphatase) whereas correct targeting of the sodium pump (a basolateral membrane protein) appeared unaffected by disruption of MTs. Few hours after drug-induced depolymerization of MTs newly synthesized apical membrane proteins appeared at the lateral cell surface. Importantly, this mistargeting of apical membrane proteins was followed by the formation of typical brush borders at the basolateral cell surface. This dramatic change in cell polarity was fully reversible after withdrawal of drugs. Basolateral brush borders were subsequently endocytosed into large vacuoles, which where then transported and incorporated into the apical cell surface. Reconstitution of cell polarity depended on the reappearance and apicobasal reorganization of the MT system.

The most likely explanation for these observations is that apically destined carrier vesicles contain a receptor for a dynein-like motor protein that may be responsible for MT-dependent transport of these vesicles to the minus end that is located underneath the apical plasma membrane. The uniform apicobasal alignment of MTs guarantees that apical carrier vesicles leaving the Golgi apparatus will be vectorially guided to the apical cell surface. As soon as MTs become depolymerized by colchicine or vinblastine, the apical carrier vesicles will loose their tracks and thus diffuse randomly throughout the cell. A fraction of these vesicles (40–60% according to [^{3}H]-fucose autoradiography) may still happen to reach the apical membrane whereas others will fuse with the basolateral membrane and thus

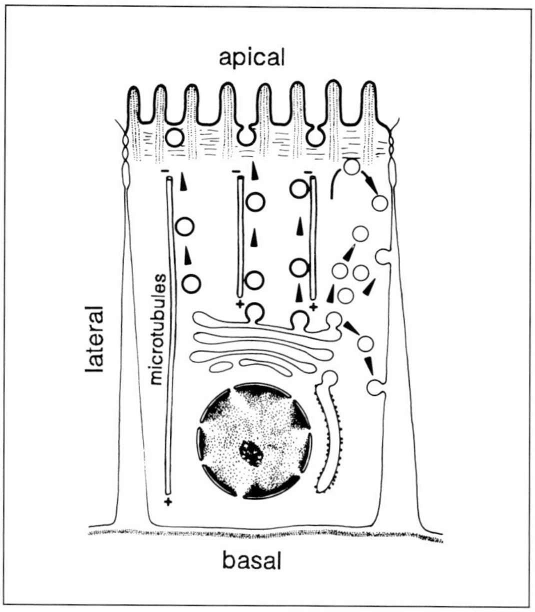

Fig. 3. Polarity and orientation of MT in the intestinal epithelium and other polarized epithelial cells. Vectorial delivery of apical membrane proteins is guaranteed by the uniform polarity of microtubules. Targeting of basolateral membrane proteins appears to be independent of microtubules. The apical terminal web may prevent basolateral membrane vesicles from apical fusion [13].

deliver apically destined proteins to the basolateral cell surface (~ 50% according to [^{3}H]-fucose autoradiography). This model demands that basolateral carrier vesicles do not associate with motor proteins and therefore follow the bulk flow of membranes that appears to be directed to the basolateral membrane domain in the intestinal epithelium [8, 9].

A central conclusion drawn from these experiments is that apical carrier vesicles can fuse with both the apical and basolateral plasma membrane whereas basolateral carrier vesicles are only able to fuse with the basolateral and not the apical membrane domain. Most likely, apical carrier vesicles are largely prevented from fusion with the basolateral domain by selective transport along MTs to the apical cell pole. Delivery of basolateral carrier vesicles to the basolateral cell surface probably does not depend on MTs, but rather appears to follow the bulk flow of membranes. At present it is not known why basolateral carrier vesicles do not fuse with the apical cell surface.

One major structural difference between the apical and basolateral membrane domain is the elaborate cytoskeleton of the terminal web that underlies the apical plasma membrane. Such an elaborate web is absent from the basolateral cell surface. Since MTs only rarely project into the terminal web the bulk of apical carrier vesicles must be able to move through this filamentous meshwork by a mechanism that is independent of MTs [15]. A possible candidate for the transport of carrier vesicles through the apical terminal web to its site of exocytosis could be myosin I (110-kD protein). Myosin I is present in the apical terminal web and in microvilli of the intestinal and kidney brush border [15], where this motor protein could mediate vesicle transport along actin filaments of the microvillus rootlets.

Association of the Kidney Sodium Pump with the Membrane Cytoskeleton

Interactions between proteins of the plasma membrane and the cytoskeleton may be important for localizing certain membrane proteins in a nonrandom fashion at specialized domains of the cell surface. The sodium pump provides an example of an integral membrane protein that is confined to the basolateral membrane surface of several polarized epithelial cells and is absent from the apical membrane [2–4]. Isoforms of ankyrin, the key protein for the linkage of the erythrocyte AE1 to the spectrin-based membrane cytoskeleton, are also confined to the basolateral membrane surface of several polarized epithelial cells including epithelial cells of the intestine and kidney tubules [16]. This observation prompted us to investigate whether the kidney sodium pump is associated with ankyrin and spectrin at the basolateral plasma membrane of kidney epithelial cells.

The first evidence for such a linkage comes from the subcellular distribution of these proteins. Ankyrin as well as the sodium pump are confined to the same microdomains of the basolateral membrane of the tubular epithelium [2]. The immunolabel is concentrated along the basal infoldings but is absent from both the flat basal membrane surface and the foot-like processes of the infoldings that abut on the basal lamina. If the sodium pump could freely diffuse in the plane of the lipid bilayer, one would expect a uniform distribution of the sodium pump along the entire basolateral cell surface rather than a restriction to specialized areas of the plasma membrane. In view of the precise colocalization of the sodium pump with ankyrin, a possible explanation for the restricted distribution of the sodium pump would be its linkage via ankyrin to the submembranous spectrin lattice, which is also

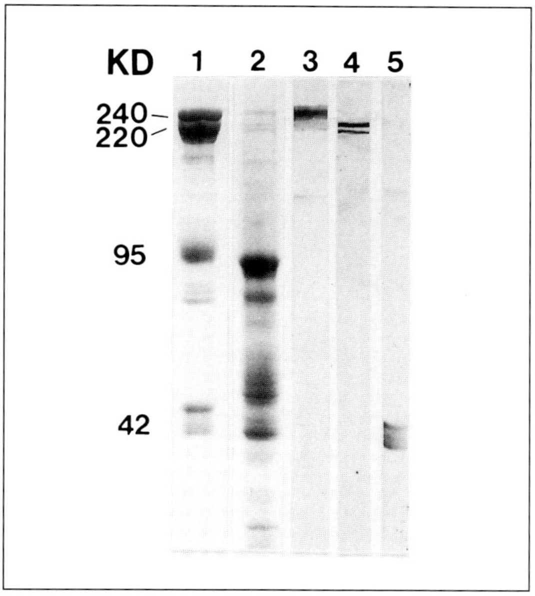

Fig. 4. SDS gel electrophoresis of purified pig parotid Na^+, K^+-ATPase demonstrating its association with spectrin, ankyrin and actin. Lane 1: Commassie blue-stained proteins of human erythrocyte membranes. Lane 2: Coomassie blue-stained lane loaded with purified Na^+, K^+-ATPase vesicles. Lanes 3–5. Immunoblot analysis of lanes corresponding to lane 2 incubated with antibodies against brain spectrin (3), erythrocyte ankyrin (4) and actin (5).

present underneath the basolateral plasma membrane in these cells [1, 16].

The second line of evidence for an association between the sodium pump and ankyrin comes from immunoprecipitation experiments in which the purified sodium pump was shown to bind erythrocyte ankyrin [2–4]. An AE1-like binding site for ankyrin appears to be likely since binding of ankyrin to the sodium pump could be inhibited in a competitive fashion by the purified cytoplasmic domain of erythrocyte AE1. Inhibition experiments with the cytoplasmic domain of AE1 indicate a binding affinity between ankyrin and the sodium pump in the range of the affinity of ankyrin for AE1 (K_D of 10^{-8} *M*).

To obtain direct proof for the tight association of the sodium pump with actin and analogs of ankyrin and spectrin in vivo we purified the sodium pump from pig kidney and pig parotid gland (two tissues particularly rich in the sodium pump) and analyzed the peripheral membrane proteins that copurify with the pump [17]. By immunoblotting and immunoprecipitation experiments direct evidence was obtained for the existence of a native complex formed between the sodium pump, actin, ankyrin and spectrin (fig. 4). Examination of the peripheral membrane proteins stripped off from sodium pump vesicles by high ionic strength showed that the pump is associated with typical double-stranded spectrin-like tetramers (100–200 μm in length). Tetramers are generally believed to represent the functional subunit of the spectrin-based membrane cytoskeleton [11].

Identification and Colocalization of AE1 and Ankyrin and Spectrin in Intercalated Cells of the Kidney Collecting Duct and Dark Cells of the Turtle Urinary Bladder

The distal nephron of the vertebrate kidney plays an important role in the regulation of the body's acid-base balance. Resorption of bicarbonate (HCO_3^-) is mediated by a subset of epithelial cells, the A type of intercalated cells which are rich in carbonic anhydrase (CA) and contain an ATP-driven H^+ pump at the apical membrane and an anion exchanger along the basolateral membrane [1, 5, 6]. Immunostaining with poly- and monoclonal antibodies specific for various epitopes of the membrane-spanning domain and of the cytoplasmic domain of AE1 localized a protein closely related to AE1 along the basolateral membrane of the CA-rich intercalated cells of the collecting duct system in the human and

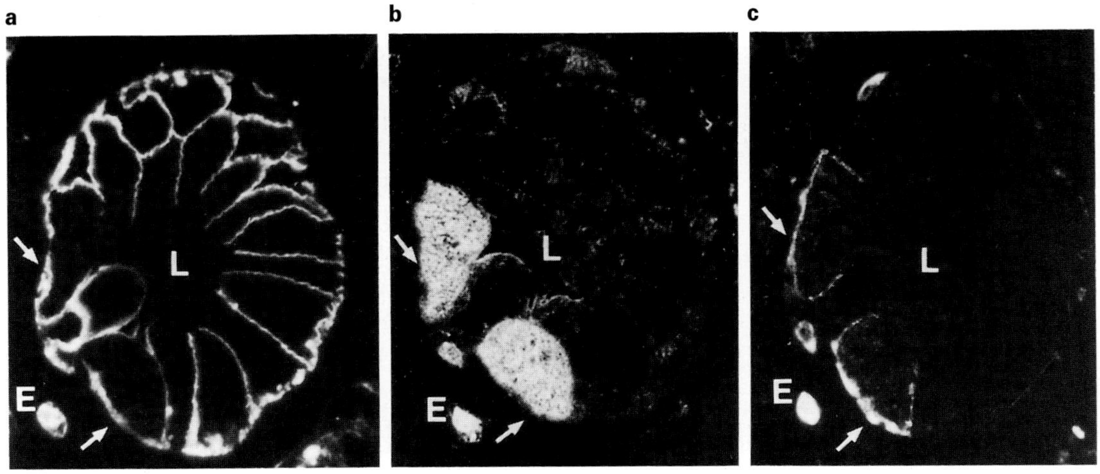

Fig. 5. Simultaneous (sequential) immunocytochemical localization of ankyrin (**a**), carbonic anhydrase I (**b**) and AE1 (**c**) in a tissue section of a medullary collecting duct of the human kidney. Note colocalization of ankyrin, carbonic anhydrase and AE1 in type A intercalated cells (arrow). L = Ductal lumen; E = erythrocyte. × 1,000.

rat kidney [1, 18] (fig. 5). The majority of dark cells of the turtle urinary bladder were also specifically stained for AE1 along the basolateral cell surface. Immunostaining with antibodies to ankyrin and spectrin revealed colocalization of these components of the membrane cytoskeleton with AE1 along the basolateral plasma membrane of intercalated and dark cells [1, 18] (fig. 5). At the ultrastructural level the immunogold label was restricted to pleated portions of the basolateral cell surface [10]. Double-labeling of kidney sections with antibodies directed against the kidney H^+-ATPase and AE1 showed that AE1 is confined to the basolateral membrane of only those intercalated cells that contain an apically located proton pump (so-called A type of intercalated cells) [19, 20].

Western blot analysis identified a major 100- to 110-kD band that was labeled with antibodies directed to various stretches of both the cytoplasmic and membrane-spanning domain of AE1 [1, 18]. Additional bands at 140 and 180 kD were only labeled with antibodies directed against portions of the membrane domain. On the other hand, no immunoreactivity was seen by immunostaining and by Western blots using three monoclonal antibodies directed to epitopes of the cytoplasmic domain as well as with an antibody directed to the N-terminal tail of 13 amino acid residues of erythroid AE1 [18, 19]. This indicates that the basolateral AE1-related anion exchanger of the kidney lacks a portion of the N-terminus of the cytoplasmic domain of erythrocyte AE1. Further confirmation of this view was obtained by polymerase chain reaction performed with cDNA from human kidney. The polymerase chain reaction products generated by various primers indicate that translation of the mRNA encoding the human kidney variant of AE1 is initiated at Met 66. Thus, human kidney AE1 probably lacks a relatively large stretch of 65 amino acids at the N-terminus [for similar findings in mice and rats, see 21 and 22]. In erythrocytes this stretch binds hemoglobin and several glycolytic enzymes, a function which may not be needed in kidney intercalated cells.

Identification of a Binding Sequence for AE1 to the Cytoskeleton

As outlined above, AE1 is linked to the spectrin-based membrane cytoskeleton by two proteins, ankyrin and protein 4.1. Since protein 4.1 is also expressed in many epithelial cells it is likely that protein 4.1 is also involved in the linkage of membrane proteins to the cytoskeleton. Although binding of ankyrin and protein 4.1 to AE1 has been well documented by in vitro binding studies it has not been possible so far to establish these interactions by defining the binding interface at the amino acid level. Comparison of the sequences of AE1 of various vertebrate species showed that the cytoplasmic domain shows only a moderate degree of homology but that it contains few highly conserved stretches. One motif (FGGLVRDIRRRY) is also expressed with negligible changes in the two nonerythroid anion exchangers (AE2, AE3) and, importantly, the C-terminal moiety of this motif occurs twice in the cytoplasmic domain of AE1 (IRRRY, LRRRY) and resembles a stretch found in the cytoplasmic tail of glycophorin A and B (IRRL), two other proteins of the erythrocyte membrane that serve as binding sites for the cytoskeleton. Binding studies between the cytoplasmic domain of AE1 and protein 4.1 showed that binding between these proteins was completely inhibited by synthetic peptides with the sequences IRRRY and LRRRY, but not by peptides with the sequence GRRRG, RRR and RIRYR [21, 22]. Antibodies and corresponding anti-idiotypic antibodies generated against the IRRRY motif also inhibited the binding of protein 4.1 to AE1. Mapping of the binding site of the anti-idiotypic antibody on protein 4.1 revealed a complementary binding motif with the sequence LEEDY [21–24].

These and other experiments allow to conclude that the binding interface between AE1 and protein 4.1 consists of a triplet of highly charged amino acid residues (IRRRY, LEEDY) that is flanked by residues with hydrophobic side chains. This combination of charged hydrophilic and uncharged hydrophobic residues may allow a two-step mechanism for binding of protein 4.1 to AE1. It is tempting to speculate that the binding sites are brought together by the forces of charge attraction. Once the charged triplets have approached each other the flanking hydrophobic residues may be close enough to bind to each other by hydrophobic interactions, which may serve to stabilize and lock the ionic binding interface between AE1 and protein 4.1.

Immunostaining with antibodies against protein 4.1 showed that protein 4.1 is also present along the basolateral surface of epithelial layers. Recent sequence data indicate that in these nonerythroid isoforms of protein 4.1 the motif identical or similar to the LEEDY binding interface (VEEDY, LEDDV, LDEEI) occurs in duplicate as does the LRRRY/IRRRY motif in AE1. We are currently investigating whether similar motifs may serve in the binding of other integral membrane proteins to the cytoskeleton.

Acknowledgements

Supported by grants of the Deutsche Forschungsgemeinschaft to Detlev Drenckhahn and Rainer Koob (SFB 286, SFB 176, Ko 808/3-2).

References

1 Drenckhahn D, Schlüter K, Allen DP, Bennett V: Colocalization of band 3 with ankyrin and spectrin at the basal membrane of intercalated cells in the rat kidney. Science 1985; 230:1287–1289.

2 Koob R, Zimmermann M, Schoner W, Drenckhahn D: Colocalization and coprecipitation of ankyrin and Na^+, K^+-ATPase in kidney epithelial cells. Eur J Cell Biol 1987;45: 230–237.

3 Nelson WJ, Veshnock PJ: Ankyrin binding to ($Na^+ + K^+$) ATPase and implications for the organization of membrane domains in polarized cells. Nature 1987;328:533–536.

4 Morrow JS, Cianci CD, Ardito T, Mann AS, Kashgarian M: Ankyrin links fodrin to the alpha subunit of Na, K-ATPase in Madin-Darby canine kidney cells and in intact renal tubule cells. J Cell Biol 1989;108: 455–465.

5 Koeppen B, Giebisch G, Malnic G: Mechanism and regulation of renal tubular acidification; in Seldin DW, Giebisch G (eds): The Kidney: physiology and Pathophysiology. New York, Raven Press, 1985, pp 1491–1525.

6 Steinmetz PR: Epithelial hydrogen ion transport; in Seldin DW, Giebisch G (eds): The Kidney: Physiology and Pathophysiology. New York, Raven Press, 1985, pp 1441–1458

7 Drenckhahn D, Oelmann M, Schaaf P, Wagner M, Wagner S: Band 3 is the basolateral anion exchanger of the dark epithelial cells of the turtle urinary bladder. Am J Physiol 1987;252:C570–C574.

8 Simons K: Membrane traffic in an epithelial cell line deried from the dog kidney. Kidney Int 1987;32: 201–207.

9 Rodriguez-Boulan E, Nelson WJ: Morphogenesis of the polarized epithelial cell phenotype. Science 1989;245:718–725.

10 Drenckhahn D, Merte C: Restriction of the human kidney band 3-like anion exchanger to specialized subdomains of the basolateral plasma membrane of intercalated cells. Eur J Cell Biol 1987;45:107–115.

11 Bennett V: The membrane skeleton of human erythrocytes and its implications for more complex cells. Annu Rev Biochem 1985;54:273–304.

12 Danielsen EM, Cowell G, Poulsen SS: Biosynthesis of intestinal microvillar proteins: Role of Golgi complex and microtubules. Biochem J 1983;216:37–42.

13 Achler C, Filmer D, Merte C, Drenckhahn D: Role of microtubules in polarized delivery of apical membrane proteins to the brush border of the intestinal epithelium. J Cell Biol 1989;109:179–189.

14 Scholey JM: Multiple microtubule motors. Nature 1990;343:118–120.

15 Drenckhahn D, Dermietzel R: Organization of the actin-filament cytoskeleton in the intestinal brush border: A quantitative and qualitative immunoelectron microscope study. J Cell Biol 1988;107:1037–1048.

16 Drenckhahn D, Bennett V: Polarized distribution of M 210000 and 190000 analogs of erythrocyte ankyrin along the plasma membrane of transporting epithelia, neurons and photoreceptors. Eur J Cell Biol 1987;43:479–486.

17 Koob R, Kraemer D, Trippe G, Aebi U, Drenckhahn D: Association of kidney and parotid Na^+, K^+-ATPase microsomes with actin and analogs of spectrin and ankyrin. Eur J Cell Biol 1990;53:93–100.

18 Wagner S, Vogel R, Lietzke R, Koob R, Drenckhahn D: Immunochemical characterization of a band 3-like anion exchanger in collecting duct of human kidney. Am J Physiol 1987;253:F213–F221.

19 Drenckhahn D, Wagner S, Jöns T, Oelmann M, Koob R: Molecular characterization of band 3-related anion exchangers in the vertebrate urinary system and Golgi apparatus; in Hamasaki N, Jennings ML (eds): Anion Transport Protein of the Red Blood Cell Membrane. Amsterdam Elsevier, 1989; pp 165–175.

20 Alper SL, Natale J, Gluck S, Lodish HF, Brown D: Subtypes of intercalated cells in rat kidney collecting duct defined by antibodies against erythroid band 3 and renal vacuolar H^+-ATPase. Proc Natl Acad Sci USA 1989;86:5429–5433.

21 Brosius FC, Alper SL, Garcia AM, Lodish HF: The major kidney band 3 gene transcript predicts an amino-terminal truncated band 3 polypeptide. J Biol Chem 1989;264:7784–7787.

22 Kudrycki KE, Shull GE: Primary structure of the rat kidney band 3 anion exchange protein deduced from a cDNA. J Biol Chem 1989; 264:8185–8192.

23 Drenckhahn D, Jöns T, Koob R, Kraemer D, Wagner S: Role of Na^+, K^+-ATPase and anion exchanger 1 (band 3) as binding sites for the cytoskeleton. Prog Cell Res 1993;2:263–268.

24 Jöns T, Drenckhahn D: Identification of the binding interface involved in linkage of cytoskeletal protein 4.1 to the erythrocyte anion exchanger. EMBO J 1992;11:2863–2867.

Renal Physiol Biochem 1993;16:15–20

Kiyoshi Kurokawa

First Department of Internal Medicine, The University of Tokyo Faculty of Medicine, Japan

Chloride Conductance of Mesangial Cells

Insights into the Transcellular Signaling of Tubuloglomerular Feedback and Its Physiological Significance

Key Words

Chloride ion
Tubuloglomerular feedback
Juxtaglomerular apparatus
Hypertension
Salt intake

Abstract

In each nephron, a change in Cl delivered to the macula densa affects afferent arteriolar tone, and thus SNGFR. This phenomenon, called tubuloglomerular feedback (TGF), is the main function of the juxtaglomerular apparatus (JGA) and serves as the fine regulator of SNGFR. The phylogeny of the JGA strongly suggests that its physiological significance may be closely related to autoregulation of RPF and GFR and that JGA and TGF will allow maintenance of SNGFR in the face of low sodium intake. We propose that JGA, which appeared from amphibia, was a prerequisite, during evolution, for transition to terrestrial life style where abundant sodium intake was not guaranteed. In other words, our nephron is in essence a salt-conserving machinery to maintain SNGFR. Further, resetting of TGF or maladaptation of TGF in the presence of abundant salt intake may underlie the pathogenesis of essential hypertension.

Introduction

Mesangial cells of the glomerulus have numerous contractile fibers similar to vascular smooth muscle cells. These characteristics of mesangial cells suggest that they contract and affect intraglomerular hemodynamics and glomerular filtration rate (GFR). It has been reported that angiotensin II (AII) causes mesangial cell contraction and thereby decreases unique values of ultrafiltration, resulting in a decrease in glomerular filtration [1, 2]. Recent advances in our knowledge of the cellular mechanisms of action of AII and of glomerular cell physiology further our understanding of the physiological properties of the mesangial cell [2]. In this report, we present our recent findings on the physiological properties of mesangial cells to advance a concept of how chloride ions (Cl^-) may function as the trans-

Kiyoshi Kurokawa
First Department of Internal Medicine
The University of Tokyo Faculty of Medicine
7-3-1 Hongo, Bunkyo-ku
Tokyo 113 (Japan)

1011–6524/93/
0162–0015 $2.75/0

cellular signal for the tubuloglomerular (TG) feedback mechanism. Further, we would like to briefly discuss our views on the physiological significance of this unique function of the nephron TG feedback.

Effects of AII on Mesangial Cell Membrane Potential

In response to brief exposure to AII the membrane potential of mesangial cells immediately and transiently depolarizes with a decrease in the input resistance [3]. Contraction of mesangial cells begins within 1 min of the application of AII, followed by membrane depolarization. This electrical response is followed by visible cell contraction which continues for several minutes. A decrease in the input resistance in response to AII indicates an increase in membrane ion permeability. The reversal potential (Vr) of the response to AII determined from the current-voltage relations prior to and at the peak of the AII-induced depolarization is about –29 mV. This value of Vr of mesangial cells strongly suggests that the opening of Cl^- channels may account for the AII-evoked membrane depolarization. Consistent with this interpretation are the data indicating that a reduction in Cl^-concentration in the incubation medium ($[Cl^-]o$) is associated with less negative Vr of the membrane depolarization. However, the measured Vr slightly deviates from the theoretical equilibrium potential of Cl^- calculated from Nernst's equation, indicating that permeability changes to other ions may also participate in the membrane depolarization. Indeed, recent observations from our laboratory using patch-clump techniques have revealed the presence of Ca^{2+}-activated nonselective cation channels and voltage-gated K^+ channels [4].

The effects of AII on mesangial cells are thought to be mediated by an increase in the concentration of intracellular Ca^{2+} ($[Ca^{2+}]i$) via inositol triphosphate (IP3] and activation of protein kinase C [5, 6]. In accordance with these postulates are the data that the Ca ionophore A23187 evoked mesangial cell contraction and the membrane potential depolarization with an increased membrane conductande, responses similar to those of AII [3]. In addition, the changes in Vr in response to A23187 with varying $[Cl^-]o$ are exactly the same as those in response to AII. These data strongly suggest that the increased Cl^- conductance by AII is mediated by an increase in $[Ca^{2+}]i$, i.e., the presence of Ca^{2+}-activated Cl^- conductance in the mesangial cell.

Extracellular Chloride Ions and Mesangial Cell Function

The presence of Cl^- conductance activated by a rise in $[Ca^{2+}]i$ and the presence of $[Cl^-]o$-dependent changes in Vr in response to AII raise the possibility that a change in $[Cl^-]o$ may modulate mesangial cellular responses to AII. A series of experiments have shown [7] (1) the percentage of mesangial cells showing unequivocal contraction in response to AII decreased from about 70 to 25% in the absence of $[Cl^-]o$ and (2) Ca^{2+} transients as well as IP_3 levels of mesangial cells in response to AII are markedly attenuated in the absence of $[Cl^-]o$. These responses of mesangial cells are similar to those evoked by exogenous PGE_2, suggesting that a reduction in $[Cl^-]o$ may simulate PGE_2 production. Indeed, PGE_2 production increased as $[Cl^-]o$ decreased. Furthermore, addition of indomethacin to the Cl^--free incubation medium prevents the attenuation of cell contraction, of Ca^{2+}-transients, and of IP_3 production by AII. These data clearly indicate that $[Cl^-]o$ is an important determinant of the mesangial function at least in part by modulating PGE_2 metabolism. It is not clear at present how a change in

[Cl–]o affects PGE_2 production by mesangial cells. The effect of [Cl^-]o may be through changes in the intracellular [Cl^-] or in cell pH. There are Na-dependent and Na-independent Cl^-/HCO^-_3 exchangers in mesangial cells, thus a change in [Cl^-]o is expected to be associated with changes in cell [Cl] and pH.

Physiological Significance of Chloride Conductance in Mesangial Cells: Implications in TG Feedback Mechanism

The presence of a unique Ca^{2+}-activated Cl^- conductance may suggest that mesangial cells may sense and respond to changes in Cl^- in their environment. In this respect, it is possible that this unique permeability of Cl^- may be important in the TG feedback system. The TG feedback mechanism is the regulation of glomerular filtration by distal tubular fluid [8, 9]. Available data suggest that a change in [Cl^-] of the fluid perfusing the macula densa segment of the early distal nephron is the critical signal for the TG feedback [8, 9]. It is thought that the primary effector mechanism involving the changes in GFR in response to alterations in distal fluid [Cl^-] are alterations in the afferent arteriolar resistance [8, 9]. Nevertheless, how a signal perceived at macula densa could be transmitted to the afferent arteriole has been poorly understood.

An important structural relationship exists between the mesangium and the juxtaglomerular apparatus. A group of interstitial cells called Goormaghtigh cells or lacis cells lie in the stalk region of the glomerulus [8]. These cells are the same kind of cells as mesangial cells, thus called extraglomerular mesangial cells. They are in close contact with macula densa cells. In addition, the lacis cells are extensively coupled with each other via gap junctions, with intraglomerular mesangial cells and with afferent arteriolar smooth muscle cells; these three types of cells, therefore, form a syncytium or, a fuctional unit [8]. It is very likely that the lacis cells are characterized by Cl^- conductance noted in the mesangial cells in our studies.

The structural and anatomical characteristics of lacis cells suggest the possibility that they may be the receptor cells which sense a change in the absorbate [Cl^-] of the macula densa cells and propagate the signal to the intraglomerular mesangial cells and to afferent arterioles. Since the interstitium-surrouding lacis cells are characterized by the lack of capillaries and lymph vessels [8], [Cl^-]o of lacis cells may be directly altered by a change in [Cl^-] in the tubular fluid perfusing macula densa. Such a change in [Cl^-]o may affect the lacis cell function which is then transmitted to the intraglomerular mesangial cells and to the afferent arterioles via gap junctions, affecting glomerular hemodynamics and filtration. It is of interest to note that Kurtz and Penner [10] recently observed that the electrophysiological response of the juxtaglomerular cells to AII is characterized by stimulation of Ca^{2+}-activated Cl^- conductance, which shows a very small unit conductance of a few pS. These responses and properties are quite similar to those observed by us in mesangial cells. These observations support our notion that these cells share some common yet unique properties which may be of fuctional significance.

Persson et al. [11] have shown that [Cl^-]o surrounding lacis cells effectively and sensitively varies in accord with a change in the luminal flow rate perfusing macula densa. It is quite likely that such a change in [Cl^-]o would be transmitted to mesangial cells and juxtaglomerular cells via gap junction. When [Cl^-] of distal fluid is reduced, [Cl^-]o around lacis cells will also decrease, so does [Cl^-]i of lacis cells. Such a change will be transmitted to the neighboring cells of this functional unit via gap junction resulting in a decrease in $[Cl^-]$i of the mesangial cells with increased PGE_2 production, decreased $[Ca^{2+}]$i, less negative Vr, and less contraction in the presence of AII. A similar directional change with a decrease in $[Cl^-]$i, will take place in the juxtaglomerular cells where smooth muscle tone may decrease due to a fall in $[Ca^{2+}]$i. In an elegant study of in vitro perfusion of the isolated juxtaglomerular apparatus, Skott and Briggs [12] have recently shown that luminal fluid $[Cl^-]$ is an important determinant of renin release from the juxtaglomerular cells. These data clearly demonstrate that a reduction in distal fluid $[Cl^-]$ stimulates renin release, and this occurs only in the presence of the intact juxtaglomerular apparatus. Because high Ca^{2+} inhibits and low Ca^{2+} stimulates renin release, these data could be interpreted as an indication of a rise in the juxtaglomerular cell $[Ca^{2+}]$i, thus relaxation of smooth muscle cells of the afferent arterioles in response to a decrease in $[Cl^-]$ perfusing macula densa. Indeed, this prediction seems correct. Itoh and Carretero [13] recently found that lowering $[Cl^-]$ perfusing macula densa results in dilation of the afferent arterioles in vitro using the isolated perfused juxtaglomerular apparatus. The events which occur in the mesangial cells, and perhaps in the lacis cells, and in the afferent arteriolar smooth muscle cells are summarized in figure 1, the original of which has been recently published [14, 15]. The schema explains our proposed mechanisms underlying the transcellular signaling in the juxtaglomerular apparatus.

Schnermann et al. [16] have proposed that adenosine may be the mediator of TG feedback. Thus, adenosine may be released in response to a change in $[Cl^-]$ reaching macula densa, which then regulates the afferent arteriolar tone. Their recent data indicate that constrictors of the afferent arteriole, angiotensin, vasopressin and probably adenosine may constrict afferent arterioles of the isolated juxtaglomerular apparatus, but fail to do so when the afferent arteriole is detached from the glomerulus [17, 18]. These data suggest that adenosine may play a permissive role and that $[Cl^-]$ at macula densa may indeed be the mediator of TG feedback through the mechanism outlined in figure 1. The data are also consistent with observations of Itoh and Carretero [13] which indicate that the afferent arteriolar tone at the entrance of the glomerulus is regulated by $[Cl^-]$ at macula densa.

Physiological Significance of Chloride Conductance in Mesangial Cells: Phylogenic Considerations

One can envision that the role of TG feedback is closely related to renal autoregulation and preservation of effective renal plasma flow in the face of changing systemic blood pressure. When renal perfusion pressure decreases, the afferent resistance decreases owing to myogenic response and, perhaps more importantly, owing to TG feedback [13, 17, 18]; this fall in afferent resistance maintains the renal plasma flow. This response is associated with a rise in AII production, which in turn constricts the efferent arteriole, allowing higher efferent resistance, and thus maintenance of intraglomerular hydraulic pressure and single nephron GFR.

An increase in $[Cl^-]$ at macula densa signals the nephron that extracellular fluid [ECF] volume may begin to decrease since both Na and Cl are the major determinants of ECF volume. In our body GFR is relatively high for the ECF volume, that is for a 60-kg man ECF volume is 12 liters and GFR is 140 liters/day. This means that every day ECF is filtered by the glomerulus more than 10 times and reabsorbed along the nephron almost completely (99%). Hence, a subtle change in NaCl handling by the kidney, particularly at distal neph-

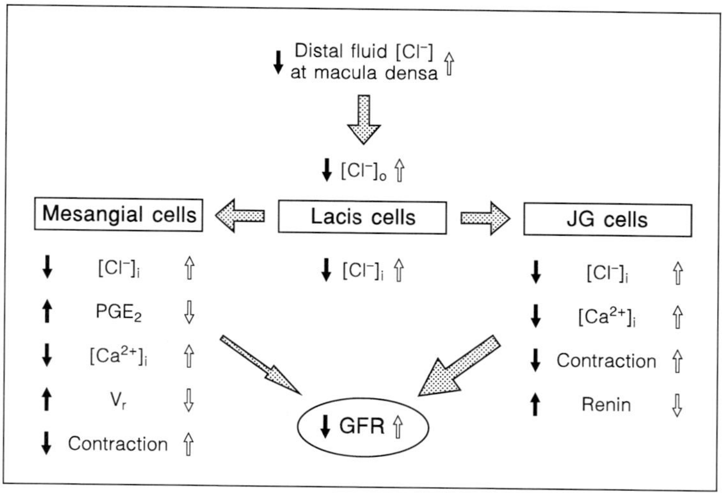

Fig. 1. Proposed model of the transcellular signaling of the TG feedback through the juxtaglomerular apparatus in response to a change in the chloride concentration perfusing macula densa. When [Cl⁻] reaching macula densa falls, [Cl⁻]o surrounding the lacis cells falls, then a decrease in [Cl⁻]i of lacis cells. This change in the [Cl⁻]i of lacis cells in then transmitted, through gap junction, to the afferent arteriolar smooth muscle cells and the intraglomerular mesangial cells. Observed and/or predicted responses of mesangial cells and afferent arteriolar smooth muscle cells are depicted in the left and right, respectively. These cellular responses will lead to an increase in single nephron GFR. The prevailing evidence suggests that the major effector of the response in the afferent arteriolar tone. See text for details, [from 14 and 15 with permission].

ron sites including the macula densa, will affect ECF volume significantly within hours. Yet, GFR must be maintained within a near-normal range to allow continuous filtration and reabsorption, the essential function of the kidney for body fluid homeostasis.

The juxtaglomerular apparatus is well developed in the amphibian, the reptile, the bird, and the mammal, and a phenomenon of TG feedback has been observed in these species. The phylogeny of the juxtaglomerular apparatus thus suggests that for these species to evolve from a NaCl-rich environment, that is the sea, to a NaCl-poor environment, that is the land, they must be endowed with a machinery to adapt very sensitively to a low NaCl intake with a varying intake of minerals and water, to maintain both the consistencies of ECF volume and composition (milieu intérieur) and of GFR to ensure the fluid and mineral homeostasis. It is not too difficult to imagine that the evolution of this machinery, the kidney, must have been essential for survival to live on the land. Stated in another way, acquisition of Cl channels in mesangial and arteriolar vascular smooth muscle cells and development of that particular structure of the juxtaglomerular apparatus have been essential for the transition from the sea to the land. We believe this is the reason for the existence of the juxtaglomerular apparatus in the nephron of these species, most of which live a terrestrial life.

Conclusions

There have been considerable advances in our understanding of physiological and biological properties of mesangial cells. Results obtained in our and other laboratories briefly outlined in this presentation may provide a reasonable explanation for the transcellular signaling through the juxtaglomerular apparatus initiated by a change in [Cl^-] perfusing macula densa. Thus, we propose that a change in luminal fluid [Cl^-] at macula densa could be transmitted through the lacis cells to the intraglomerular mesangial cells and to the afferent arteriole including juxtaglomerular cells by virtue of the unique anatomical structure of the juxtaglomerular apparatus and of the presence of Cl^- conductance in mesangial, juxtaglomerular, and probably in lacis cells. We hope that this working hypothesis, though highly speculative, will be of value in elucidating the cellular and transcellular mechanisms underlying the tubuloglomerular feedback. Such particular function and structure of the juxtaglomerular apparatus may be explained by considering its evolution, that is, it is the critical mechanism to assure both near-normal ECF volume and high GFR while on a poor NaCl intake.

References

1 Dworkin LD, Ichikawa I, Brenner BM: Hormonal modulation of glomerular function. Am J Physiol 1983;244:F95–F104.

2 Mene P, Simonson M, Dunn MJ: Physiology of the mesangial cell. Physiol Rev 1989;69:1348–1424.

3 Okuda T, Yamashita N, Kurokawa K: Angiotensin II and vasopressin stimulate calcium activated chloride conductance in rat mesangial cells. J Clin Invest 1986;78:1443–1447.

4 Matsunaga H, Yamashita N, Miyajima Y, Okuda T, Chang H, Ogata E, Kurokawa K: Ion channel activities of cultured rat mesangial cells. Am J Physiol 1991;261:F808–F814.

5 Bonventre JV, Skorecki KL, Kreisberg JI, Cheung JY: Vasopressin increases cytosolic free calcium concentration in glomerular mesangial cells. Am J Physiol 1986;251: F94–F102.

6 Hassid A, Pidikiti N, Gamero D: Effects of vasoactive peptides on cytosolic calcium in cultured mesangial cells. Am J Physiol 1986;251: F1018–F1028.

7 Okuda T, Kojima I, Ogata E, Kurokawa K: Extracellular Cl^- ions modify rat mesangial cell contraction by modulating cell inositol triphosphate and Ca^{++} via enhanced prostaglandin E2. J Clin Invest 1989;84: 1866–1872.

8 Schnermann J, Briggs JP: Function of the juxtaglomerular apparatus: Local control of glomerular hemodynamics; in Seldin DW, Giebisch G (eds): The Kidney: Pysiology and Pathophysiology. New York, Raven Press, 1985, pp 665–697.

9 Briggs JP, Schnermann J: The tubuloglomerular feedback mechansim: Functional and biochemical aspects. Annu Rev Physiol 1987;49: 251–273.

10 Kurtz A, Penner R: Angiotensin II induces oscillations of intracellular calcium and blocks anomalous inward rectifying potassium current in mouse renal juxtaglomerular cells. Proc Natl Acad Sci USA 1989;86: 3423–3427.

11 Persson BE, Sakai T, Marsh DJ: Juxtaglomerular interstitial hypertonicity in *Amphiuma:* Tubular origin-TGF signal. Am J Physiol 1988; 254:F445–F449.

12 Skott O, Briggs JP: Direct demonstration of macula densa mediated renin secretion. Science 1987;237: 1618–1620.

13 Itoh S, Carretero QA: An in vivo approach to the study of macula densa-mediated glomerular hemodynamics. Kidney Int 1990;38: 1206–1210.

14 Kurokawa K, Okuda T: Calcium activated chloride conductance of mesangial cells. Kidney Int 1990; 38(suppl 30):S48–S50.

15 Kurokawa K, Okuda T; Chloride conductance of mesangial cells; in Koide H, Endou H, Kurokawa K (eds): Cellular and Molecular Biology of the Kidney. Contrib Nephrol. Basel, Karger, 1991, vol 95, pp 76–81.

16 Schnermann J, Weihprecht H, Briggs J: Inhibition of tubuloglomerular feedback during adenosine$_1$ receptor blockade. Am J Physiol 1990;258:F553–F561.

17 Weihprecht H, Lorenz JN, Briggs JP, Schnermann J: Vasoconstrictive effect of angiotensin and vasopressin in isolated rabbit afferent arterioles. Am J Physiol 1991;261: F273–F282.

18 Briggs JP, Lorenz JN, Weihprecht H, Schnermann J: Purinergic receptors on renal afferent arterioles (abstract). J Am Soc Nephrol 1991;2: 501.

Renal Physiol Biochem 1993;16:21–36

Eberhard Schlatter

Physiologisches Institut,
Albert-Ludwigs-Universität
Freiburg, BRD

Regulation of Ion Channels in the Cortical Collecting Duct

Key Words
K^+ channel
Na^+ channel
Cl^- channel
pH dependence
Principal cell

Abstract
Properties of ion channels of the cortical collecting duct (CCD) and their relevance for the macroscopic conductances are discussed. Although the regulation of the Na^+ conductance by various hormones is widely studied, the relevant Na^+ channel appears to be extremely difficult to be detected in the intact preparation. Three different K^+ channels with slope conductances of about 30, 140 and 80 pS (excised, 145 mmol/l KCL and 145 mmol/l NaCl on both sides of the membrane) have been found in principal cells of the CCD so far. The first two channels are located in the luminal, the latter one in the basolateral membrane. The two luminal channels are highly sensitive to the cytosolic pH and are also inhibited by cytosolic ATP. The small luminal K^+ channel, highly active on the cell, is most likely responsible for K^+ secretion. The large luminal K^+ channel is involved in the volume regulation. The basolateral K^+ channel, again highly active on the cell, is probably responsible for the recirculation of K^+ across this membrane. The physiological role of the observed Cl^- channels is still unknown.

Transport in the Cortical Collecting Duct

The cortical collecting duct (CCD) of the mammalian kidney is responsible for transepithelial reabsorption of Na^+, Cl^-, and HCO_3^- and secretion of K^+, NH_4^+, and H^+. Together with the reabsorption of water these transport processes allow a fine adjustment of urinary excretion of these solutes in accordance with the needs of the organism. Three different cell types – principal cells, α-cells, and β-cells – are involved in these transport processes which are regulated by hormones and other factors such as cellular pH. A large number of original studies and excellent reviews exists on the

Priv. Doz. Dr. Eberhard Schlatter
Physiologisches Institut
Albert-Ludwigs-Universität
Hermann-Herder-Strasse 7
D-W-7800 Freiburg (FRG)

1011–6524/93/
0162–0021 $2.75/0

regulation of the water permeability in the CCD by adiuretin (ADH) [1, 2]. In the last few years we learned that in addition to its hydroosmotic effect ADH also increases Na^+ and K^+ transport [3–9]. Isoproterenol, via cAMP, stimulates the transport of Cl^- and HCO_3^- [10–12] in this nephron segment. Regulation of Na^+ and K^+ transport in this nephron segment by aldosterone is another well studied issue [13–15].

Some electrolyte transport processes in the CCD are directly or indirectly coupled, such as Na^+ reabsorption and K^+ secretion and K^+ and H^+ secretion. Transport of the first two ions occurs via the same cell, the principal cell, and coupling is due to electrical coupling of Na^+ uptake and K^+ secretion across the luminal membrane. Therefore, when Na^+ reabsorption increases K^+ secretion increases as well. K^+ secretion, however, decreases, when H^+ secretion is enhanced for example during acidosis. Because K^+ and H^+ are at least to a large portion transported via different cell types, principal and intercalated cells, the coupling must be indirect, possibly via changes in cellular pH.

Principal cells are responsible for Na^+ reabsorption and at least most of the K^+ secretion [8]. The energy-consuming process for the transport of these two electrolytes is provided by the basolateral Na^++K^+-ATPase [3, 16, 17]. The only significant entry mechanism for Na^+ across the luminal membrane is the Na^+ conductance in this membrane [3, 5]. K^+ secretion in these cells occurs via a K^+ conductance in the luminal membrane, while a portion of the K^+ which is taken up by the Na^++K^+-ATPase recycles across the basolateral K^+ conductance [3, 9, 17, 18]. In the rabbit, however not in the rat, the basolateral membrane of principal cells has a large Cl^- conductance [17, 18]; its contribution to transepithelial Cl^- transport, however, is still unclear. In the rat, principal cells do not participate in transepithelial Cl^- reabsorption [19].

This review will focus on the regulation of ion conductances of principal cells of the CCD. It will summarize properties of the macroscopic conductances and describe ion channels found in the CCD and attempt a correlation of the two.

Methods to Study Ion-Conductances and Channels in the CCD

Several methodological approaches have been used during the last few years to study ion conductances and ion channels of the CCD from rat and rabbit kidneys: (1) ion flux measurements [5–7, 16], (2) microelectrode impalements with conventional and ion-selective electrodes [3, 17–19], (3) patch clamp studies of single channel and whole-cell currents [20–27], and (4) measurements of intracellular Ca^{2+} activity and cellular pH [28–32]. All these methods were applied to the intact in vitro perfused isolated CCD [3, 28], the cut open tubule [21], freshly isolated CCD cells [33], or CCD cells in culture [34–36]. Figure 1 shows a cartoon of three of these methods, microelectrode impalements in the isolated perfused tubule, patch clamp studies in the intact isolated CCD, and patch clamp studies on freshly isolated CCD cells. Data obtained with these methods in the author's laboratory will be discussed and supplemented by observations obtained by other laboratories with similar methods.

Na^+ Conductance of Principal Cells of CCD

Na^+ reabsorption by principal cells of the CCD is mediated via basolateral Na^++K^+-ATPase and a luminal amiloride-sensitive Na^+ conductance [3, 5]. This Na^+ conductance is hormonally controlled by aldosterone and

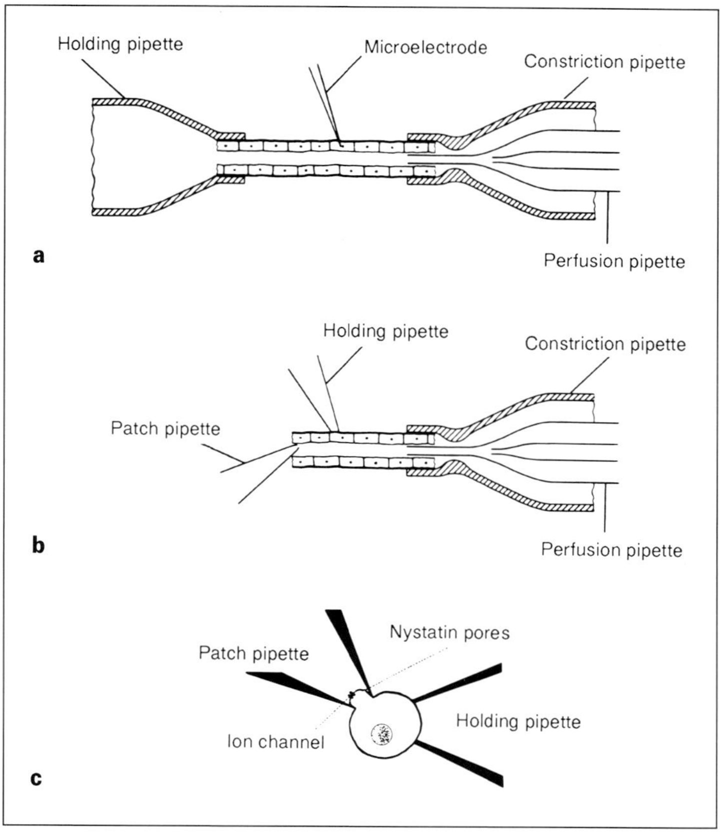

Fig. 1. Cartoon of methods used to study the regulation of ion conductances and ion channels in the CCD. **a** Isolated in vitro perfused CCD segment with microelectrode to record membrane voltage and fractional resistance of individual cells. **b** Isolated in vitro perfused CCD segment with patch-clamp electrode advanced into the tubular lumen to record ion channel activity from the luminal membrane. **c** Cell-attached nystatin or slow whole-cell recording of membrane voltage, membrane or cellular conductance and single channel activity of freshly isolated CCD cells.

ADH [5, 6, 37, 38]. Aldosterone leads to a slowly acting and long-lasting increase in Na^+ reabsorption via an increase in Na^+ conductance, activity of the Na^++K^+-ATPase, and K^+ conductance by both activation of existing and synthesis of new transport systems [14, 15, 39]. ADH acutely activates the Na^+ conductance via a cAMP-mediated mechanism [26, 40]. Figure 2 shows, that transepithelial voltage and conductance of rat CCD increase with ADH and are decreased by low concentrations of the Na^+ channel blocker amiloride. These transepithelial effects of ADH are paralleled by a depolarization (ADH) and a hyperpolarization (amiloride) of the voltage of a principal cell. ADH depolarizes these cells by activating Na^+ channels in the luminal membrane [3], thus increasing Na^+ reabsorption, which can be completely inhibited by amiloride [5]. This increase in the Na^+ conductance by ADH is more pronounced when Na^+ reabsorption is stimulated by aldosterone, thus both hormones act synergistically [3, 5, 9, 33]. Figure 3 depicts an original recording of the membrane voltage of a freshly isolated principal cell of rat CCD measured with a patch-clamp electrode in the slow whole-cell configuration. Already 0.1 μmol/l amiloride significantly hyperpolarizes this cell indicating a significant Na^+ conductance. When the K^+ conductance of this cell is reduced by 1 mmol/l Ba^{2+}, added to the bath, the hyperpolarization induced by amiloride is markedly increased.

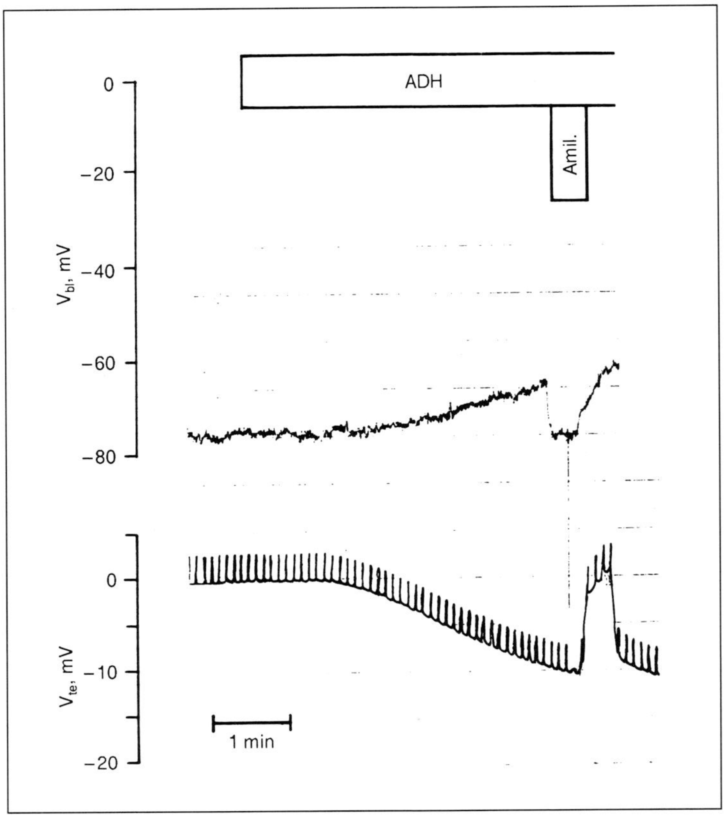

Fig. 2. Original recording of the transepithelial voltage (V_{te}) of an isolated perfused rat CCD segment and of the basolateral membrane voltage (V_{bl}) of a principal cell. ADH (200 pmol/l) increases V_{te} and depolarizes V_{bl}, whereas amiloride (Amil., 10 μmol/l) has opposite effects. These responses indicate the activation and inhibition of a Na^+ conductance by these maneuvers.

Na^+ Channels in Rat CCD

Identification of the Na^+ channel responsible for Na^+ uptake across the luminal membrane of principal cells and the examination of its properties in the intact CCD have been extremely difficult. Only few observations have been published so far [23, 41]. This Na^+-selective channel has a conductance of only 5–10 pS when recorded on the cell with 140 mmol/l Na^+ in the patch pipette [23]. This channel seems to be regulated by cytosolic pH, acidification decreasing its activity, and indirectly by the cytosolic Ca^+ activity. Increasing Ca^{2+} activity reduces channel activity [41]. Figure 4 shows original current traces and the current/voltage relation of such a channel recorded from freshly isolated CCD cells of the rat. A similar Na^+ channel is observed more frequently in cultured CCD or A6 cells [42–44]. The difficulty in demonstrating this Na^+-selective channel in the intact CCD, even under conditions where the Na^+ conductance is maximally stimulated by aldosterone and ADH, may indicate that the described channel is not the relevant Na^+ channel for Na^+ reabsorption in the CCD. There might be another type of Na^+ channel, which has an even smaller single channel conductance and thus cannot be resolved with classical patch clamp methods.

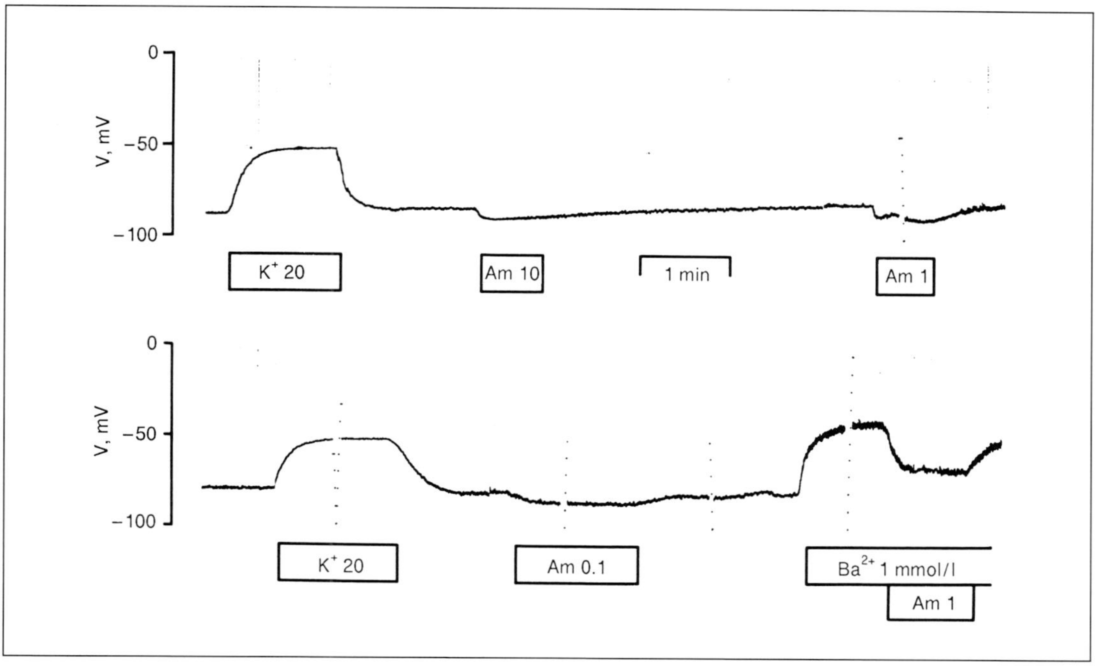

Fig. 3. Original recording of the membrane voltage (V) of a freshly isolated principal cell of rat CCD. Effects of a K^+ concentration step from 3.6 to 18.6 mmol/l, of amiloride (Am, 0.1–10 μmol/l), and of Ba^{2+} (1 mmol/l). Note the significant hyperpolarization of V already with 0.1 μmol/l amiloride and the largely increased amiloride effect in the presence of Ba^{2+}.

K^+ Conductances of Principal Cells of CCD

K^+ secretion in the CCD occurs predominantly across principal cells and is driven by the activity of the basolateral Na^++K^+-ATPase. K^+ leaves the cell conductively across both the basolateral and the luminal membrane [3, 17, 18]. In the rat CCD the basolateral membrane of principal cells is only conductive to K^+ [3], whereas in the rabbit the basolateral membrane has a large Cl^- conductance in parallel to the K^+ conductance [17, 18]. Figure 3 shows in addition to the amiloride effect (see above) the depolarization of the membrane voltage of a freshly isolated principal cell of rat CCD by an increase in the extra-cellular K^+ concentration from 3.6 to 18.6 mmol/l. Addition of Ba^{2+} (1 mmol/l) strongly depolarizes this cell. Both effects and the high negative voltage of this cell indicate the presence of a large K^+ conductance in principal cells of rat CCD.

In many epithelial cells the K^+ conductance is functionally coupled to the activity of the Na^++K^+-ATPase [45]. This is also true for principal cells of rat CCD as is indicated in figure 5. The depolarization of the basolateral membrane voltage of principal cells of isolated perfused CCD segments is reduced after inhibition of the Na^++K^+-ATPase by ouabain. When, however, the Na^++K^+-ATPase is stopped because Na^+ entry across the luminal membrane is inhibited by amiloride the K^+

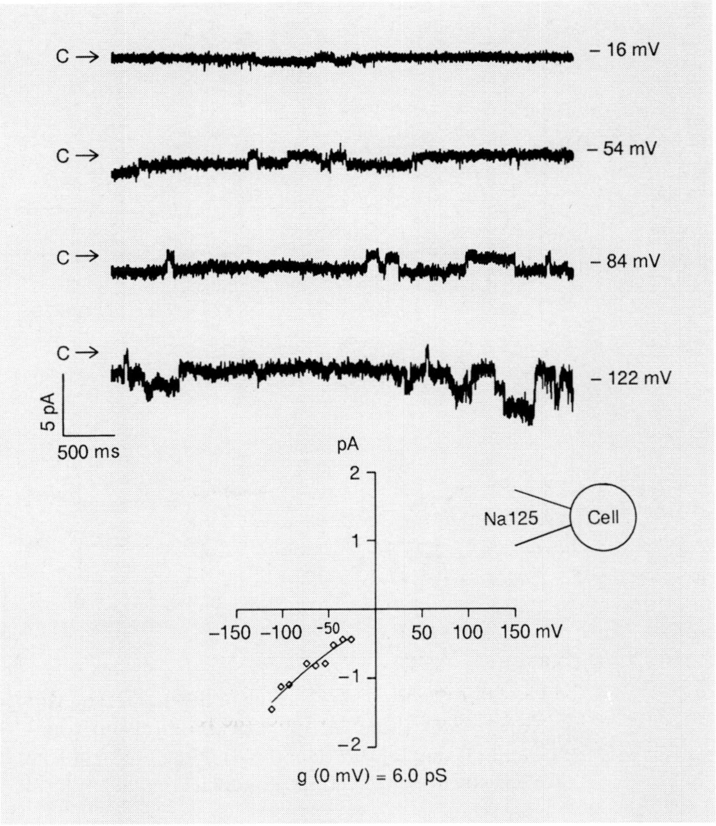

Fig. 4. Typical current traces of a small conductance Na^+ channel of a freshly isolated principal cell of rat CCD. The lower part shows the current/voltage relation of this channel, which has an estimated slope conductance at 0 mV of 6 pS. Voltages are clamp voltages applied in addition to the membrane potential. C indicates the closed state of the channel.

concentration step-induced depolarization is as large as under control conditions. This phenomenon could be explained by a direct or indirect regulation of the K^+ conductance by changes in the cellular Ca^{2+} activity. When the Na^++K^+-ATPase is inhibited by ouabain Na^+ will still enter the cell via the luminal Na^+ conductance resulting in an increased cytosolic Na^+ activity. In the other situation, when Na^+ entry via the luminal Na^+ conductance is inhibited, the Na^++K^+-ATPase will continue to transport Na^+ out of the cell until a minimal Na^+ activity is reached in the cell and the pump stops. The difference in the cytosolic Na^+ activity may lead to changes in the cytosolic Ca^{2+} activity via Na^+/Ca^{2+} exchange. A high cytosolic Na^+ activity will decrease, a low cytosolic Na^+ activity will increase cytosolic Ca^{2+} activity. Such changes in the Ca^{2+} activity could change the activity of Ca^{2+}-dependent K^+ channels directly or the activity of Ca^{2+}-independent K^+ channels via changes in the Ca^{2+}-dependent protein kinase C activity. The latter has been demonstrated for the small conductance K^+ channel in the luminal membrane of rat CCD [46].

The macroscopic K^+ conductance of principal cells is inhibited by the K^+ channel blocker Ba^{2+}, by verapamil and by the presence of extracellular NH_4^+ [47]. The K^+ conductance of the luminal membrane is inhibited by extracellular NH_4^+ as well. Such an inhibition of K^+ conductances in the presence of extracellular NH_4^+ is most likely due to NH_4^+

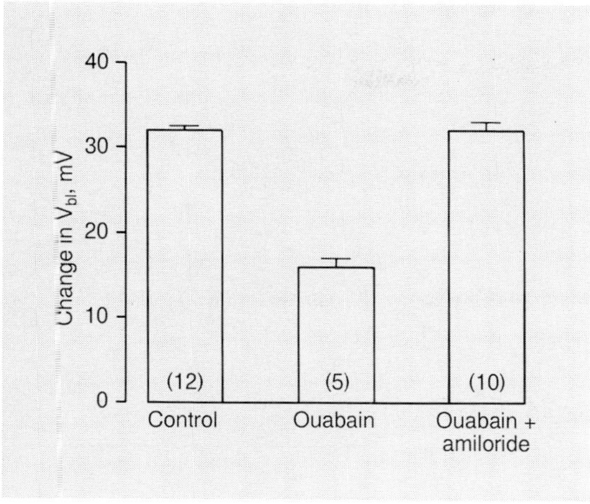

Fig. 5. Effect of ouabain (0.5 mmol/l) and amiloride (10 μmol/l) on the depolarization of the basolateral membrane voltage (V_{bl}) of principal cells from isolated perfused CCD segments of the rat induced by an elevation of the basolateral K^+ concentration from 3.6 to 18.6 mmol/l. Note that direct inhibition of the Na^++K^+-ATPase by ouabain, however, not by indirect inhibition of pump activity by amiloride reduces the K^+ concentration step-induced depolarization of V_{bl}, i.e. the K^+ conductance of the basolateral membrane.

ions entering principal cells followed by a cytosolic acidification and inhibition of pH-sensitive K^+ channels [47]. Changes in the K^+ secretion via principal cells probably depend mostly on changes in the driving force for K^+ across the luminal membrane [9]. An additional increase in the K^+ conductance of the luminal membrane by hormones has been demonstrated for aldosterone [15, 37, 38], but appears less likely for ADH [9]. Both hormones stimulate K^+ secretion [6, 7, 16] independently of changes in the K^+ conductance just by the depolarization of principal cells due to an increase in the luminal Na^+ conductance induced by these hormones initially [3, 33]. The increase in the Na^+ conductance by both hormones probably exceeds that of the K^+ conductance because the voltage of principal cells depolarizes under these conditions, whereas it should hyperpolarize if the change in the K^+ conductance was larger than that in the Na^+ conductance. On the other hand, K^+ channels in the luminal membrane of principal cells of rat CCD have been shown to be regulated by cAMP-dependent protein kinase A [48, 49] (see below).

K^+ Channels in Principal Cells of CCD

Several K^+ channels with different properties have been described from isolated CCDs, from freshly isolated CCD cells, and from CCD cells in culture. The selectivity properties, the influence of various inhibitors, as well as the regulation of channel activity by a number of cytosolic factors have been examined for these channels. This information helps to judge the physiological role of these different K^+ channels for the principal cell of the CCD.

Large Conductance K^+ Channel of the Luminal Membrane

Initially a large conductance K^+ channel was described for the luminal membrane of principal cells of rat CCD [21, 22], which has a unitary conductance of 140 pS when studied under cell-free conditions with high NaCl and high KCl solutions on the two sides of the membrane, respectively. The open probability of this channel is high under those cell-free conditions, however, extremely rare when it is studied on the cell. This discrepancy is probably due to its strong dependence on the cytosolic Ca^{2+} activity, with a significant activation of the channel at cytosolic Ca^{2+} activities of above 1 μmol/l [21, 22, 28]. Figure 6 demonstrates the Ca^{2+} dependence of this maxi-K^+ channel. As is typical for this Ca^{2+}-dependent large conductance K^+ channel its open probability is also dependent on the voltage applied across the membrane. This is demonstrated in figure 7. At normal hyperpolarized

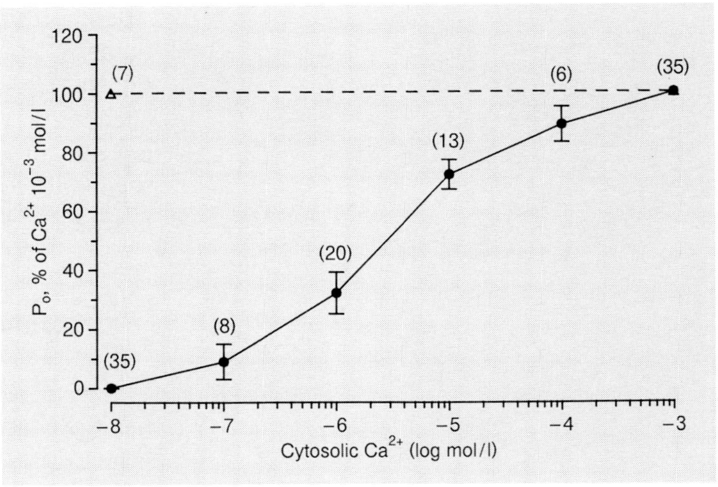

Fig. 6. Ca^{2+} dependence of the open probability (P_O) for the large conductance K^+ channel (——) and the small conductance K^+ channel (– – –) in the luminal membrane of principal cells of rat CCD. Data are obtained from inside-out patches with 145 mmol/l K^+ in the pipette and 145 mmol/l Na^+ in the bath. Numbers in parentheses indicate the number of observations.

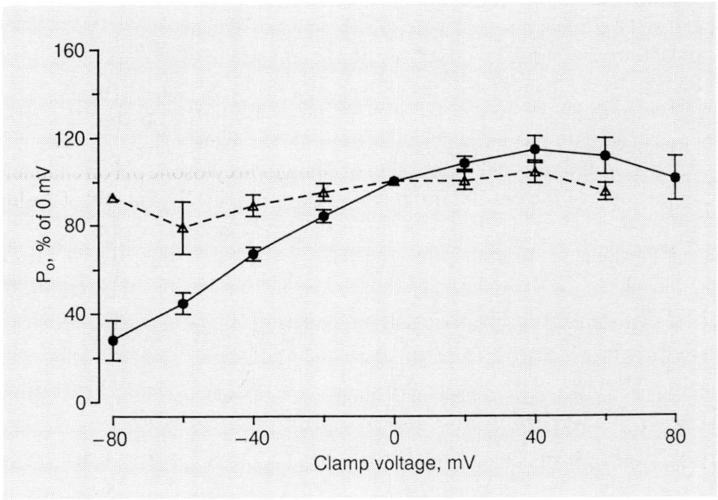

Fig. 7. Voltage dependence of the open probability (P_O) for the large conductance K^+ channel (——; n = 52) and the small conductance K^+ channel (– – –; n = 16) in the luminal membrane of principal cells of rat CCD. Data are obtained from inside-out patches with 145 mmol/l K^+ in the pipette and 145 mmol/l Na^+ in the bath. Note the activation of the large channel by depolarization and the voltage independence of the small channel.

membrane voltages this channel is poorly active, but its activity increases with membrane depolarizations. This voltage- and Ca^{2+}-dependent maxi-K^+ channel was also found in apical membranes of intercalated cells [50] and of cultured rabbit principal cells [34, 36]. Again in these cells the activity of this channel on the cell is close to zero.

When studied in the excised configuration with 1 mmol/l Ca^{2+} in the bathing solution (i.e. on the cytosolic surface of the membrane) this channel is insensitive to changes in the cytosolic pH up to alterations of almost 1 pH unit (fig. 8). Addition of ATP at a concentration up to 3 mmol/l with a high Ca^{2+} activity on the cytosolic side of the channel is also without effect (fig. 9) [28]. When this channel, however, is exposed to a Ca^{2+} activity of 1 μmol/l on its cytosolic surface, both acidification and increases in the ATP concentration downreg-

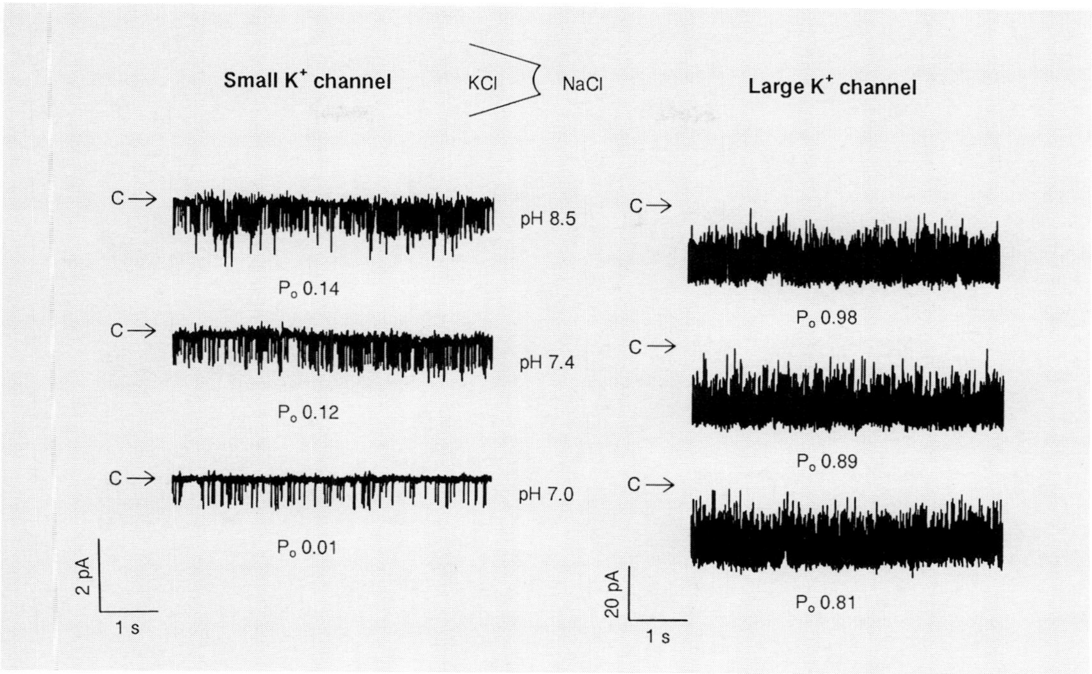

Fig. 8. Effect of changes in cytosolic pH on channel activity in excised inside-out patches of the small (left) and the large (right) K^+ channel of the luminal membrane of principal cells of rat CCD. Bath solution (i.e. on the cytosolic side of the membrane) contains 1 mmol/l Ca^{2+}. Open probability (P_O) is sampled over a period of at least 1 min. C indicates the closed state of the channel.

ulate the open state probability [28]. This is demonstrated with original current traces depicted in figure 10. The absence of the regulation by these two factors in the presence of a high cytosolic Ca^{2+} activity may be due to the maximal stimulation of channel activity under this condition.

The large conductance K^+ channel of the luminal membrane of rat CCD has a selectivity sequence of $p_K > p_{Rb} > p_{NH_4} > p_{Cs} = P_{Li} = P_{Na} = p_{choline} = 0$. As is characteristic for the maxi-K^+ channel from other preparations and other epithelial K^+ channels [51], the conductance sequence for this channel differs from the selectivity sequence: $g_K > g_{NH_4} > g_{Rb} > g_{Li} = g_{choline} > g_{Cs} = g_{Na} = 0$. In addition, high concentrations of NH_4^+, Rb^+, and Cs^+ inhibit the K^+ current through this channel [20]. This channel is also inhibited by a large number of compounds like Ba^{2+} (half-maximal inhibition, IC_{50}, at 30 µmol/l), TEA^+ (IC_{50} = 400 µmol/l), quinine (IC_{50} = 120 µmol/l), and quinidine (IC_{50} = 220 µmol/l). As we know meanwhile various K^+ channels are also blocked by the Ca^{2+} channel blockers verapamil and diltiazem [51]. This is also the case for this K^+ channel (IC_{50} = 7 and 120 µmol/l for verapamil and diltiazem, respectively). Like other maxi-K^+ channels, this K^+ channel from the CCD is sensitive towards the venom from scorpion charybdotoxin and is insensitive towards the venom from bee apamin [20].

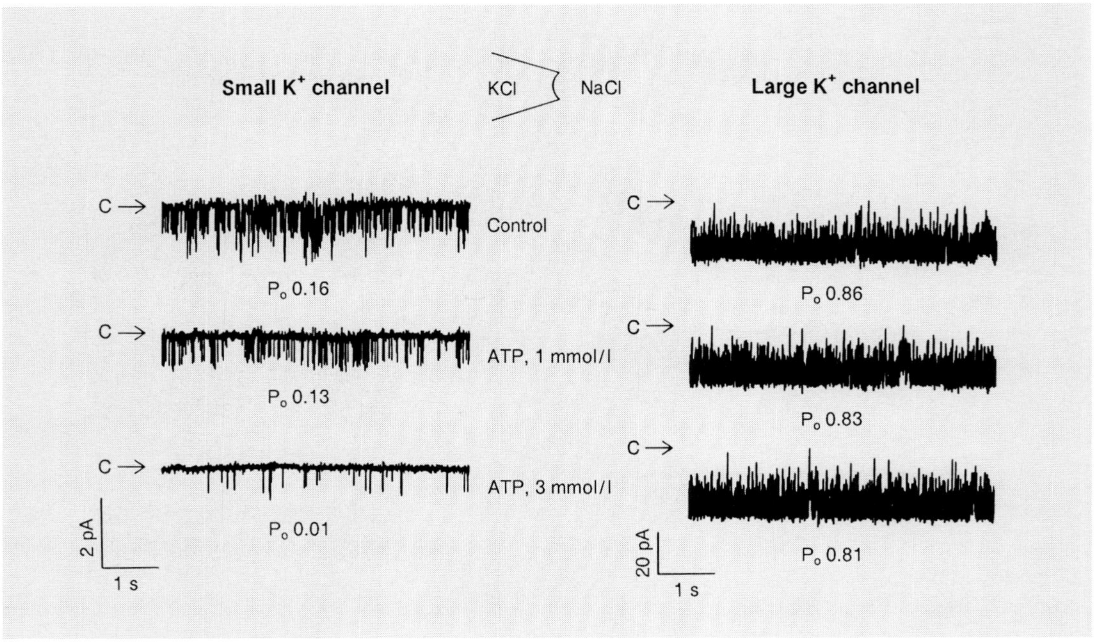

Fig. 9. Effect of changes in cytosolic ATP concentration on channel activity in excised inside-out patches of the small (left) and the large (right) K^+ channel of the luminal membrane of principal cells of rat CCD. Bath solution (i.e. on the cytosolic side of the membrane) contains 1 mmol/l Ca^{2+}. Open probability (P_O) is sampled over a period of at least 1 min. C indicates the closed state of the channel.

The voltage and Ca^{2+} dependence of this channel explain its extremely low activity when the cell is at normal hyperpolarized membrane voltage with low cytosolic Ca^{2+} activities. Thus, it was concluded, that this maxi-K^+ channel does not contribute to the K^+ secretion in the CCD. An increase in cytosolic Ca^{2+} by agonists such as high concentrations of ADH [52] or eicosanoids [53] may, however, activate this channel and thus increase K^+ secretion.

Recently it was demonstrated that this maxi-K^+ channel is activated in principal cells of the CCD, when the cells are osmotically swollen [28, 53]. Such an activation of channel activity is shown in figure 11 for a freshly isolated principal cell of rat CCD. This activation by hypotonic cell swelling is mediated by an increase in the intracellular Ca^{2+} activity (fig. 12). The Ca^{2+} increase under these conditions is mostly due to an influx of extracellular Ca^{2+}, as removal of extracellular Ca^{2+} prevents the swelling-induced increase in cytosolic Ca^{2+} activity [28, 53].

A contribution of this maxi-K^+ channel in the luminal membrane of principal cells to K^+ secretion in the CCD may only be significant when cells are strongly depolarized by an activation of the luminal Na^+ conductance and/or by an agonist-induced increase in cytosolic Ca^{2+} activity. Its predominant physiological role, however, appears to be an increase in the pathway for K^+ extrusion out of the cell as a volume regulatory response after cell swelling.

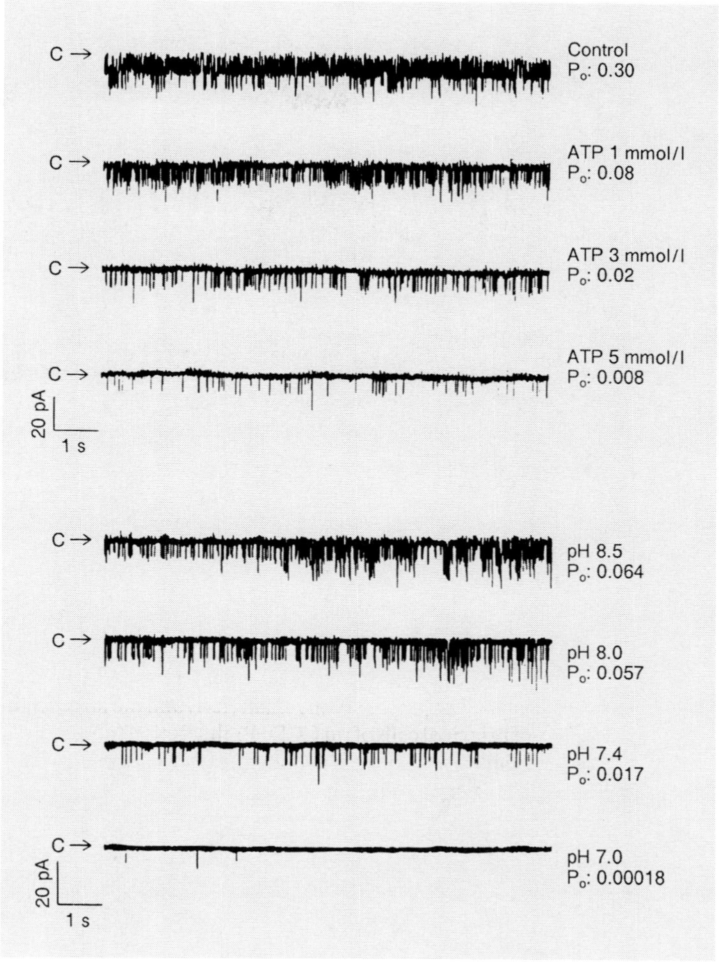

Fig. 10. Effect of changes in cytosolic ATP concentration (top 4 traces) and in cytosolic pH (bottom 4 traces) on channel activity in excised inside-out patches of the large conductance K^+ channel of the luminal membrane of principal cells of rat CCD. Now bath solution (i.e. on the cytosolic side of the membrane) only contains 1 μmol/l Ca^{2+}. Open probability (P_O) is sampled over a period of at least 1 min. C indicates the closed state of the channel.

Small Conductance K^+ Channel of the Luminal Membrane

On the cell a small conductance K^+ channel is found in the luminal membrane with very high activity. This channel is independent on the cytosolic Ca^{2+} activity (see fig. 6) and its open probability is not altered by changes in the membrane voltage (see fig. 7). This small K^+ channel shows rectification when studied on the cell with a high K^+ concentration in the patch clamp electrode. Under such conditions it has an inward conductance of 35 pS and an outward conductance of 15 pS [24, 27, 33]. Its high activity on the cell in normally hyperpolarized principal cells makes this channel the most likely candidate for the pathway for K^+ secretion via principal cells of CCD.

Changes in the cytosolic pH alter the activity of this channel, again acidification is leading to a decrease of the open probability of the channel and an alkalinization is activating channel activity (see fig. 8) [27]. In addition to the regulation of this small conductance K^+ channel by pH, it is regulated by cytosolic ATP (see fig. 9). Concentrations of ATP above 0.1 mmol/l inhibit its activity [48]. Low

11
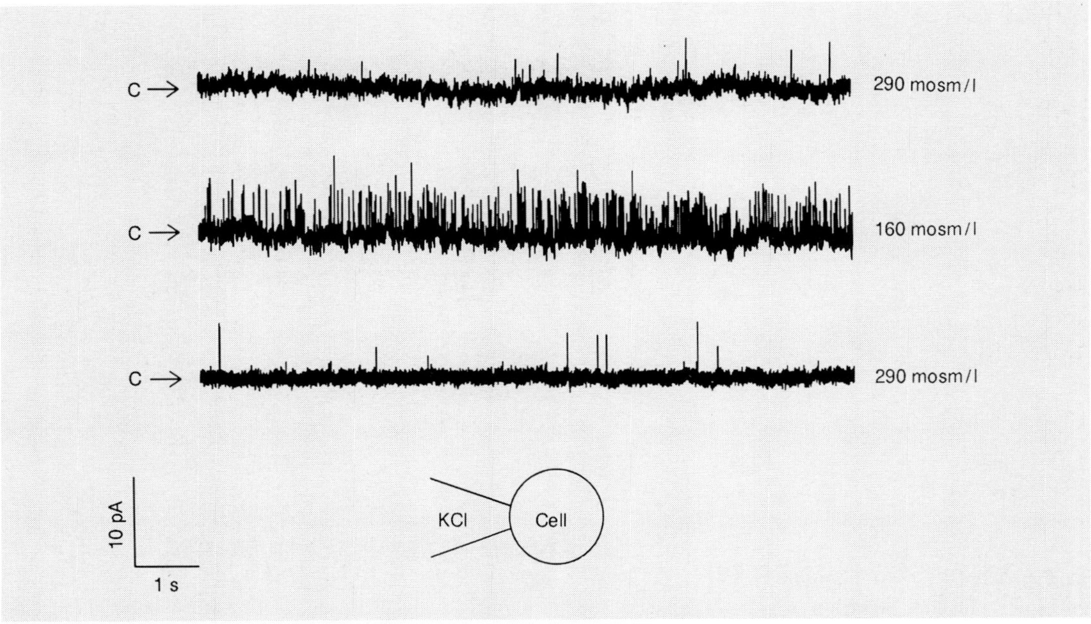

12
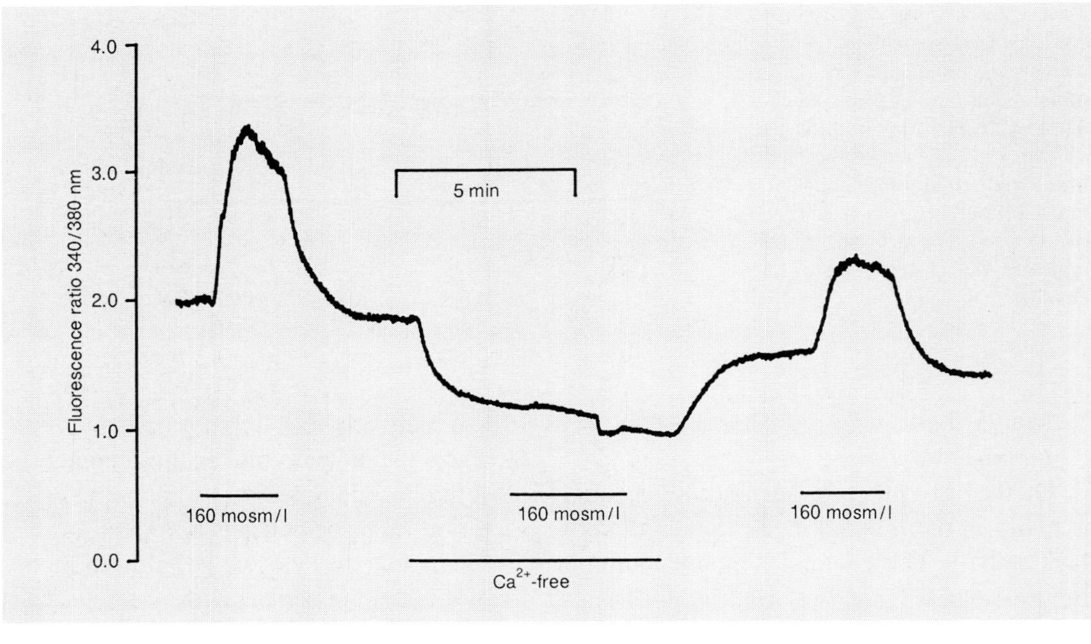

Fig. 11. Activation of the large conductance K^+ channel by hypotonic cell swelling (reduction in extracellular osmolarity from 290 to 160 mosm/l) of a freshly isolated principal cell of rat CCD. Cell-attached nystatin recording. C indicates the closed state of the channel.

Fig. 12. Effect of hypotonic cell swelling (reduction in extracellular osmolarity from 290 to 160 mosm/l) on the cytosolic Ca^{2+} activity (measured with FURA-2 as fluorescence ratio at 340 and 380 nm) of freshly isolated CCD cells of the rat. Swelling-induced rise in internal Ca^{2+} disappears in the absence of extracellular Ca^{2+}.

concentrations of cytosolic ATP, however, are necessary to activate this channel via protein kinase A-mediated phosphorylation [48]. Protein kinase C or arachidonic acid downregulate the channel activity [49, 54]. This complex regulation system of the small conductance K^+ channel in the luminal membrane of principal cells allows variations in transepithelial K^+ secretion by various hormones involving separate cellular transduction pathways.

In addition, the strong pH dependence of this channel presents an easy explanation for the observed decrease in K^+ secretion during acidosis. The similar strong pH dependence of the large conductance K^+ channel and the small conductance K^+ channel in the luminal membrane of principal cells results in a parallel up- or downregulation of both K^+ channels with changes in pH in conditions when the maxi-K^+ channel is activated as well.

Recently, a dependence of this small conductance K^+ channel on the activity of the basolateral Na^++K^+-ATPase has been demonstrated [46]. Inhibition of the Na^++K^+-ATPase by removing extracellular K^+ downregulates the luminal K^+ channel activity. This downregulation seems to involve Ca^{2+}-dependent protein kinase C as signal transduction pathway (see above).

K^+ Channels in the Basolateral Membrane of CCD

The identification and examination of ion channels in the basolateral membrane of renal tubules is difficult because of the inaccessibility of this membrane for patch clamp studies due to the basement membrane. First, small K^+ channels from the basolateral membrane with a conductance of 2–20 pS have been found in a preparation of isolated CCD segments with mechanically ruptured basement membranes [55]. The described channel has a very low activity at normal hyperpolarized membrane voltages and it is activated by strong membrane depolarization.

Recently, in the author's laboratory a K^+ channel of intermediate conductance (80 pS) with high activity on the cell was identified in mildly collagenase-treated CCDs [56]. Figure 13 depicts an example of this channel, showing original current traces recorded on the cell and the respective current/voltage relation. This channel is also pH-sensitive. These properties are very comparable to those of the K^+ channel described in the luminal membrane of rat thick ascending limb [51] of similar size.

Cl^- Channels in Principal Cells of CCD

In the rabbit CCD the principal cell has a Cl^--conductive basolateral membrane, thus suggesting that Cl^- transport may occur via these cells. In the rat, however, there is no evidence for Cl^- transport systems in principal cells whatsoever [19]. So far Cl^--selective channels have only been described for the basolateral membrane of rabbit CCD [57] or the luminal membrane of principal cells in cultures from rabbit CCD [58]. The basolateral Cl^- channel has a slope conductance of 46 pS with a high open probability on the cell and, thus, it is considered to be responsible for the macroscopic Cl^- conductance of this membrane. The contribution of the three different Cl^- channels observed in the luminal membrane of rabbit principal cells to transepithelial Cl^- transport remains unclear. In addition, little is known about the selectivity properties, the regulation and the pharmacological alteration of these channels.

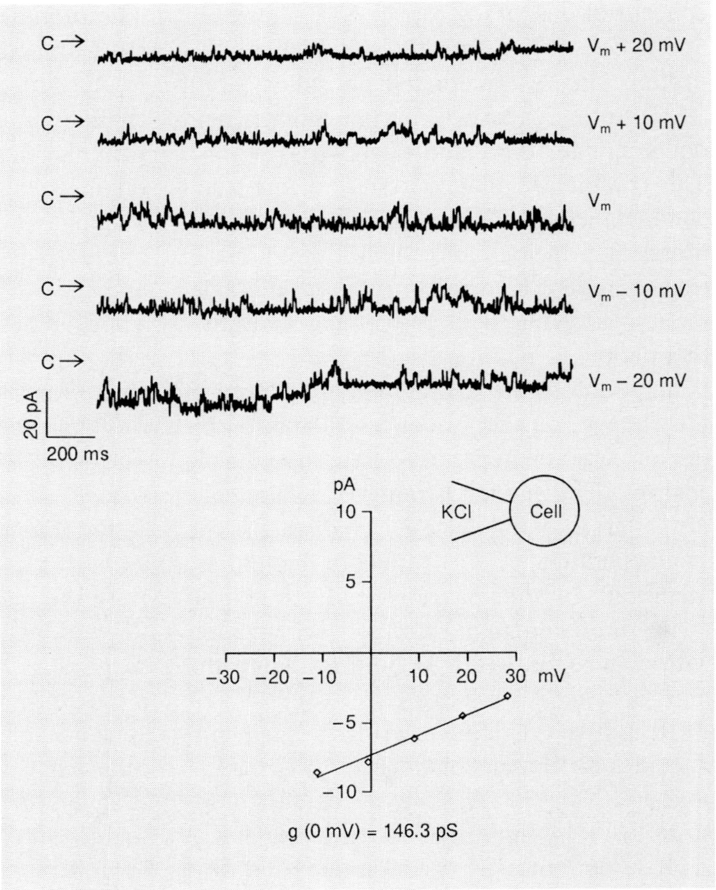

Fig. 13. K^+ channel recorded from the basolateral membrane of an isolated collagenase-treated CCD segment of the rat. The upper part shows typical current traces at different clamp voltages which were applied on top of the membrane voltage of this cell-attached recording. The slope conductance of this channel with 145 mmol/l K^+ in the pipette at 0 mV was 146 pS. C indicates the closed state of the channels.

Conclusion

The principal cell of the mammalian CCD has predominant K^+ conductances in both membranes. Two different channels are well described for the luminal membrane: a smaller one, which is the channel responsible for normal and hormonally activated K^+ secretion, and a larger one, which is activated when principal cells are swollen and possibly when cells are strongly depolarized and have an elevated cytosolic Ca^{2+} activity. Especially the small conductance K^+ channel shows a complex regulation by various transduction pathways and cytosolic factors. Information on the K^+ channels of the basolateral membrane is just coming up. All three K^+ channels are pH-sensitive. This pH dependence provides an attractive explanation for the observed coupling between K^+ secretion and H^+ secretion in this nephron segment.

Although we understand the regulation of the macroscopic Na^+ conductance of principal cells of CCD fairly well, our knowledge about the relevant Na^+ channel is quite limited. The question of the relevance for transepithelial Cl^- transport of the observed Cl^- conductance and Cl^- channel in rabbit CCD is again completely unresolved.

Acknowledgements

I gratefully acknowledge the technical assistance of Mrs. I. Burhoff, A. Hauser, S. Haxelmans, and J. Siebert during the work in the author's laboratory. Data presented from the author's laboratory were obtained in collaboration with Prof. Dr. R. Greger, Dr. M. Bleich and J. Hirsch. I thank Prof. Dr. R. Greger for his careful reading of the manuscript. Work quoted from the author's laboratory was supported by Deutsche Forschungsgemeinschaft Schl 277/2-1 to 2-3.

References

1 Harris HW, Jr, Strange K, Zeidel ML: Current understanding of the cellular biology and molecular structure of the antidiuretic hormone-stimulated water transport pathway. J Clin Invest 1991;88:1–8.
2 Verkman AS: Water channels in cell membranes. Annu Rev Physiol 1992;54:97–108.
3 Schlatter E, Schafer JA: Electrophysiological studies in principal cells of rat cortical collecting tubules. ADH increases the apical membrane Na^+-conductance. Pflügers Arch 1987;409:81–92.
4 Reif MC, Troutman SL, Schafer JA: Sustained response to vasopressin in isolated rat cortical collecting tubule. Kidney Int 1984;26:725–732.
5 Reif MC, Troutman SL, Schafer JA: Sodium transport by rat cortical collecting tubule. Effects of vasopressin and desoxycorticosterone. J Clin Invest 1986;77:1291–1298.
6 Tomita K, Pisano JJ, Knepper MA: Control of sodium and potassium transport in the cortical collecting duct of the rat. Effects of bradykinin, vasopressin and deoxycorticosterone. J Clin Invest 1985;76:132–136.
7 Schafer JA, Troutman SL: Effect of ADH on rubidium transport in isolated perfused rat cortical collecting tubules. Am J Physiol 1986;250: F1063–F1072.
8 Schlatter E: Antidiuretic hormone regulation of electrolyte transport in the distal nephron. Renal Physiol Biochem 1989;12:65–84.
9 Schafer JA, Troutman SL, Schlatter E: Vasopressin and mineralocorticoid increase apical membrane driving force for K^+ secretion in rat CCD. Am J Physiol 1990;258:F199–F210.
10 Schuster VL: Cyclic adenosine monophosphate-stimulated anion transport in rabbit cortical collecting duct. Kinetics, stoichiometry, and conductive pathways. J Clin Invest 1986;78:1621–1630.
11 Dietl P, Schwiebert E, Stanton BA: Cellular mechanisms of chloride transport in the cortical collecting duct. Kidney Int 1991;40(suppl 33): S125–S130.
12 Dietl P, Kizer N, Stanton BA: Conductive properties of a rabbit cortical collecting duct cell line: Regulation by isoproterenol. Am J Physiol 1992;262:F578–F582.
13 Morel F, Doucet A: Hormonal control of kidney functions at the cell level. Physiol Rev 1986;66:377–468.
14 Young DB: Quantitative analysis of aldosterone's role in potassium regulation. Am J Physiol 1988;255: F811–F822.
15 Oberleithner H: Acute aldosterone action in renal target cells. Cell Physiol Biochem 1991;1:2–12.
16 Schafer JA, Troutman SL: Potassium transport in cortical collecting tubules from mineralocorticoid-treated rat. Am J Physiol 1987;253: F76–F88.
17 Koeppen BM, Biagi BA, Giebisch G: Intracellular microelectrode characterization of the rabbit cortical collecting duct. Am J Physiol 1983;244:F35–F47.
18 O'Neil RG, Sansom SC: Electrophysiological properties of cellular and paracellular conductive pathways of the rabbit cortical collecting duct. J Membr Biol 1984;82:281–295.
19 Schlatter E, Greger R, Schafer JA: Principal cells of cortical collecting ducts of the rat are not a route of transepithelial Cl^- transport. Pflügers Arch 1990;417:317–323.
20 Schlatter E, Bleich M, Hirsch J, Markstahler U, Fröbe U, Greger R: Cation specificity and pharmacological properties of the Ca^{2+} dependent K^+ channel of rat cortical collecting ducts. Pflügers Arch, 1993, in press.
21 Hunter M, Lopes AG, Boulpaep EL, Giebisch G: Regulation of single potassium ion channels from apical membrane of rabbit collecting tubule. Am J Physiol 1986;251: F725–F733.
22 Frindt G, Palmer LG: Ca-activated K channels in apical membrane of mammalian CCT, and their role in K secretion. Am J Physiol 1987; 252:F458–F467.
23 Palmer LG, Frindt G: Amiloride-sensitive Na channels from the apical membrane of the rat cortical collecting tubule. Proc Natl Acad Sci USA 1986;83:2767–2770.
24 Frindt G, Palmer LG: Low-conductance K channels in apical membrane of rat cortical collecting tubule. Am J Physiol 1989;256:F143–F151.
25 Geibel J, Zweifach A, White S, Wang W, Giebisch G: K^+ channels of the mammalian collecting duct. Renal Physiol Biochem 1990;13:59–69.

26 Frindt G, Sackin H, Palmer LG: Whole-cell currents in rat cortical collecting tubule: Low-Na diet increases amiloride-sensitive conductance. Am J Physiol 1990;258: F562–F567.
27 Wang W, Schwab A, Giebisch G: Regulation of small-conductance K^+ channel in apical membrane of rat cortical collecting tubule. Am J Physiol 1990;259:F494–F502.
28 Hirsch J, Leipziger J, Fröbe U, Schlatter E: Regulation and possible physiological role of the Ca^{2+}-dependent K^+-channel of cortical collecting ducts of the rat. Pflügers Arch, 1993, in press.
29 Hébert RL, Jacobson HR, Breyer MD: Prostaglandin E_2 inhibits sodium transport in rabbit cortical collecting duct by increasing intracellular calcium. J Clin Invest 1991;87: 1992–1998.
30 Naruse M, Uchida S, Ogata E, Kurokawa K: Endothelin 1 increases cell calcium in mouse collecting tubule cells. Am J Physiol 1991;261: F720–F725.
31 Dagher G, Sauterey C: Regulation of intracellular pH in rabbit cortical connecting tubule and cortical collecting duct. Biochim Biophys Acta 1991;1133:17–24.
32 Silver RB, Frindt G, Palmer LG: Regulation of principal cell pH by Na/H exchange in rabbit cortical collecting tubule. J Membr Biol 1992;125:13–24.
33 Schlatter E, Fröbe U, Greger R: Ion conductances of isolated cortical collecting duct cells. Pflügers Arch 1992;421:381–387.
34 Gitter AH, Beyenbach KW, Christine CW, Gross P, Minuth WW, Frömter E: High-conductance K^+ channel in apical membranes of principal cells cultured from rabbit renal cortical collecting duct anlagen. Pflügers Arch 1987;408:282–290.
35 Light DB, Schwiebert EM, Fejes-Tóth G, et al: Chloride channels in the apical membrane of cortical collecting duct cells. Am J Physiol 1990;258:F273–F280.
36 Ling BN, Hinton CF, Eaton DC: Potassium permeable channels in primary cultures of rabbit cortical collecting tubule. Kidney Int 1991; 40:441–452.
37 O'Neil RG, Helman SI: Transport characteristics of renal collecting tubules: Influences of DOCA and diet. Am J Physiol 1977;233:F544–F558.
38 Schwartz GJ, Burg MB: Mineralocorticoid effects on cation transport by cortical collecting tubules in vitro. Am J Physiol 1978;235:F576–F585.
39 Garty H: Mechanisms of aldosterone action in tight epithelia. J Membr Biol 1986;90:193–205.
40 Schafer JA, Troutman SL: cAMP mediates the increase in apical membrane Na^+ conductance produced in rat CCD by vasopressin. Am J Physiol 1990;259:F823–F831.
41 Palmer LG, Frindt G: Effects of cell Ca and pH on Na channels from rat cortical collecting tubule. Am J Physiol 1987;253:F333–F339.
42 Hamilton KL, Eaton DC: Single-channel recordings from amiloride-sensitive epithelial sodium channel. Am J Physiol 1985;249:C200–C207.
43 Marunaka Y, Eaton DC: Effects of vasopressin and cAMP on single amiloride-blockable Na channels. Am J Physiol 1991;260:C1071–C1084.
44 Ling BN, Hinton CF, Eaton DC: Amiloride-sensitive sodium channels in rabbit cortical collecting tubule primary cultures. Am J Physiol 1991;261–F933–F944.
45 Schultz SG: Homocellular regulatory mechanisms in sodium-transporting epithelia: Avoidance of extinction by 'flush-through'. Am J Physiol 1981;241:F579–F590.
46 Wang W, Geibel J, Giebisch G: The modullary mechanisms of the apical low-conductance K^+ channel of rat CCD during inhibition of the basolateral Na^+-K^+-ATPase. Am J Physiol, 1993, in press.
47 Schlatter E, Lohmann E, Greger R: Properties of the potassium conductance of principal cells of rat cortical collecting ducts. Pflügers Arch 1992;420:39–45.
48 Wang W, Giebisch G: Dual effect of adenosine triphosphate on the apical small conductance K^+ channel of the rat cortical collecting duct. J Gen Physiol 1991;98:35–61.
49 Wang W, Giebisch G: Dual modulation of renal ATP-sensitive K^+ channel by protein kinases A and C. Proc Natl Acad Sci USA 1991;88: 9722–9725.
50 Pácha J, Frindt G, Sackin H, Palmer LG: Apical maxi K channels in intercalated cells of CCT. Am J Physiol 1991;261:F696–F705.
51 Bleich M, Schlatter E, Greger R: The luminal K^+ channel of the thick ascending limb of Henle's loop. Pflügers Arch 1990;415:449–460.
52 Ando Y, Breyer MD, Jacobson HR: Dose-dependent heterogenous actions of vasopressin in rabbit cortical collecting ducts. Am J Physiol 1989;256:F556–F562.
53 Ling BN, Webster CL, Eaton DC: Eicosanoids modulate apical Ca^{2+}-dependent K^+ channels in cultured rabbit principal cells. Am J Physiol 1992;263:F116–F126.
54 Wang W, Cassola A, Giebisch G: Arachidonic acid inhibits the secretory K^+ channel of cortical collecting duct of rat kidney. Am J Physiol 1992;262:F554–F559.
55 Sansom SC, Agulian S, Muto S, Illig V, Giebisch G: K activity of CCD principal cells from normal and DOCA-treated rabbits. Am J Physiol 1989;256:F136–F142.
56 Hirsch J, Schlatter E: An intermediate-conductance K^+-channel in the basolateral membrane of rat cortical collecting duct (CCD). Pflügers Arch, 1993, in press.
57 Sansom SC, La B-Q, Carosi SL: Double-barreled chloride channels of collecting duct basolateral membrane. Am J Physiol 1990;259:F46–F52.
58 Christine CW, Laskowski FH, Gitter AH, Beyenbach KW, Gross P, Frömter E: Anion channels in the apical membrane of collecting duct principal cells in culture. Cell Physiol Biochem 1991;1:76–88.

Renal Physiol Biochem 1993;16:37–47

J. Biber
H. Murer

Institute of Physiology,
University of Zürich, Switzerland

Towards a Molecular View of Renal Proximal Tubular Reabsorption of Phosphate

Key Words
Phosphate transport
Proximal tubule

Abstract
Apical sodium-dependent transport of inorganic phosphate (P_i) in the proximal tubule plays a crucial role in renal P_i reabsorption and consequently in the maintenance of P_i homeostasis. This transport system represents a main target for acute and long-term regulation such as by parathyroid hormone, by growth factors and dietary intake of phosphate. In this short review we briefly describe the currently established cellular mechanism of proximal tubular P_i reabsorption and its regulation via the apical Na/P_i cotransport system. In a second part we will outline recent progress made with respect to the molecular cloning of renal Na/P_i cotransport systems. Knowledge about the molecular identity of these transport systems will make it possible to resolve yet unanswered questions about the molecular mechanisms involved in the physiology of the regulation of renal P_i reabsorption.

Introduction

As a site of output the kidney plays a central role in controling and maintaining the level of the extracellular concentration of inorganic phosphate (P_i). Renal handling of phosphate can be considered approximately as the product of glomerular filtration and proximal tubular reabsorption since P_i which is almost freely filtered in the glomeruli is reabsorbed to a large extent (up to 80%) along the proximal tubule; reabsorption and regulation of P_i in distal parts of the nephron seem likely but have been poorly described. A large number of observations indicate that the proximal tubule also represents a main target for the physiological regulation of renal P_i handling [for reviews, see 1–5]. The cellular mechanisms of proximal tubular transepithelial P_i transport and its regulation by many hormon-

Dr. J. Biber
Institute of Physiology
University Zürich-Irchel
Winterthurerstr. 190
CH–8057 Zürich (Switzerland)

1011–6524/93/
0162–0037 $2.75/0

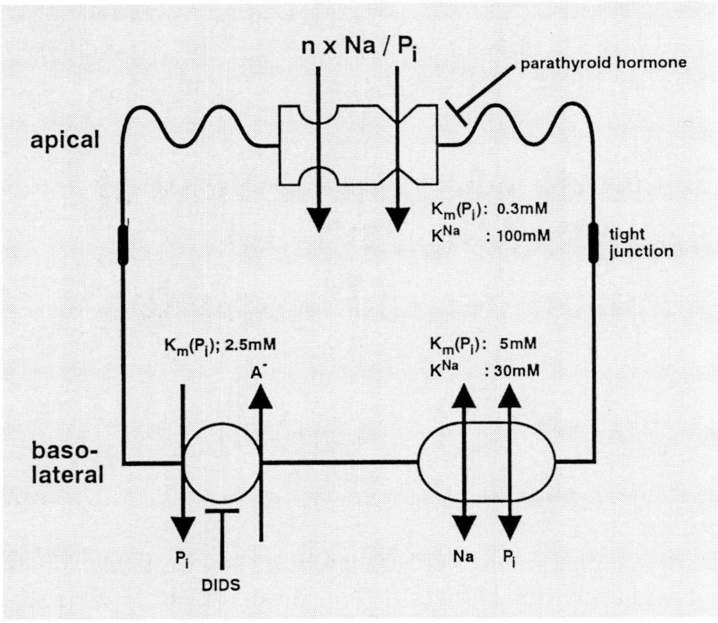

Fig. 1. Current model of proximal tubular transepithelial transport of P_i. The details of the single steps are discussed in the text. Cytosolic interactions of P_i, such as with gluconeogenesis and oxidative phosphorylation, are not included in this model.

al and nonhormonal factors have been described in microperfusion studies using isolated tubular preparations, by experiments using isolated brush-border and basolateral membranes and in studies performed with various established renal epithelial cell lines [for reviews, see 4–7]. Alltogether, these studies demonstrated that the first step of proximal tubular P_i reabsorption occurs via an apically localized sodium-dependent transport system for phosphate and that this Na/P_i cotransport mechanism plays a major role in the physiological control of renal P_i reabsorption. Thus to understand the molecular details of the mechanisms of the regulation of renal P_i reabsorption it would be important to know the molecular identity of proximal tubular apical Na/P_i cotransport systems.

In this review we briefly summarize our current knowledge about the cellular mechanisms of proximal tubular P_i reabsorption and expose the work that is presently in progress to identify renal Na/P_i cotransport systems with the aim to elucidate the molecular mechanisms involved in the regulation of renal P_i reabsorption.

Cell Physiology of Renal P_i Reabsorption

Transmembrane Movements of P_i in the Proximal Tubule

Apical Entry step. A schematic model of proximal tubular transepithelial P_i transport is shown in figure 1. This model has been deduced from a variety of studies using isolated proximal tubules (microperfusion studies), isolated plasma membrane (brush-border and basolateral) vesicles and established renal epithelial cell cultures. It is important to note that the presented model does not take into account a possible existence of an inter- and intranephron heterogeneity of proximal tubular apical Na/P_i cotransport systems (see below). Additionally, this model does not include metabolic interactions of cytosolic P_i, as for example with gluconeogenesis.

In early microperfusion studies P_i reabsorption in the proximal tubule has been shown to be obligatory dependent on the presence of luminal sodium [8, 9]: Since P_i reabsorption can be inhibited by ouabain transcellular transport of P_i represents a secondary active transport process which is driven by the apically inwardly directed gradient of sodium maintained by the basolaterally localized Na/K-ATPase. A direct link between an inwardly directed gradient of sodium and P_i transport has been demonstrated with brush border membrane vesicles isolated from rat kidney [10]. The basic characteristics of apical Na/P_i cotransport described in these early studies have since been confirmed in many studies using brush-border membrane vesicles isolated from kidneys of different mammals and with various established renal epithelial cell lines [cited in 4, 6].

Based on the interaction of P_i and Na ions the Na/P_i cotransport can be characterized as follows. The apparent K_m value for P_i lies in the range of 100–300 μ*M* and the apparent K_m for Na interaction lies between 70 and 100 m*M*. The stoichiometry exceeds unity, under physiological conditions most likely 1 PO_4^{2-} ion is cotransported together with 2 Na^+ ions. Thus at neutral pH values the system operates in a electroneutral manner; a contribution of the membrane potential for optimal P_i reabsorption can however not be excluded [4]. Based on several observations, such as (1) sigmoidal dependence of P_i transport on Na concentration, (2) increase of Na increases the affinity for P_i and (3) affinity for Na does not seem to be saturated at physiological Na concentrations, a glide symmetry model has been proposed [6]. Alternatively, a model of random binding has also been proposed [11]; at physiological concentrations of P_i and Na, however, the two kinetic models might not differ.

From a thermodynamic point of view (assuming an inside-negative potential of –65 mV [12]) passive distribution of P_i across the apical membrane would result in an approximately 10- to 100-fold lower intracellular concentration of P_i as compared to the extracellular (luminal) one. This however would be in contrast to the intracellular P_i concentration which lies between 0.7 and 1.8 m*M* as measured by ^{31}P-NMR [13]. On the other hand, if one assumed a stoichiometry of 2 Na ions per 1 P_i for apical Na/P_i cotransport and an inwardly directed gradient of sodium in the order of 10:1, the steady state concentration of P_i would results in an intracellular accumulation of P_i by a factor of 100. Based on the most likely intracellular concentration of free P_i of around 1 m*M*, this then would mean that the intracellular concentration of P_i is kept far above its passive (electrochemical) distribution but far below its thermodynamic equilibrium. This situation strongly suggests that the apical entry step via a Na/P_i cotransport system exceeding a stoichiometry of unity might represent an ideal target for physiological regulation. As the driving forces seem to be far in excess, regulation of the apical entry step could be envisaged by an alteration of the number of (active) apical Na/P_i cotransport systems or by altering the kinetic properties of individual transport systems.

Basolateral Exit Step. Exit of P_i across the basolateral membrane occurs along its electrochemical gradient. Contraluminal P_i transport has been investigated with intact tubular preparations and isolated basolateral membrane vesicles; however, P_i transport through the basolateral membrane is poorly understood. As illustrated in figure 1, there is evidence that P_i leaves the cell via two different P_i transport systems. Based on experiments with isolated basolateral membranes and intact tubular preparations there is evidence for a sodium-independent DIDS-sensitive anion exchange mechanisms possibly involving bicarbonate ions [14, 15]; this transport mechanisms does not seem to transport sulfate. In addition, a Na-dependent transport pathway for P_i has been demonstrated with basolateral membranes isolated from dog kidney [16] and a cultured renal epithelial cell line (OK cells) [17]. In contrast to the apical Na/P_i cotransport, Na-dependent transport of P_i through the basolateral membrane is characterized by a low K_m value for P_i (millimolar range) and a stoichiometry of 1:1 [6, 17].

Heterogeneity of P_i Transport Systems. As illustrated in figure 1 at least three different transmembranous P_i transport pathways have to be considered in the transport of P_i across the proximal tubular epithelial cell. Additionally to this intracellular multiplicity of P_i transport mechanisms evidence was obtained for the existence of an intranephron heterogeneity as well as for an internephron heterogeneity between cortical and juxtamedullary proximal tubules. Evidence for the later two heterogeneities arose from experiments performed with brush-border membrane vesicles isolated from different cortical regions. In brush-border membrane vesicles isolated from rat kidney cortex a system of low capacity and high affinity (for P_i) and one system of high capacity and low affinity was demonstrated [18]. Na/P_i cotransport systems of different capacities have also been described in brush-border membrane vesicles isolated from outer cortical and outer medullary cortex of the pig and rat [19–21].

So far, no experimental evidence has been reported on a possible heterogeneity of basolateral P_i transport mechanisms. Due to experimental difficulties of preparing basolateral membranes, this question will most likely not be resolved until basolateral P_i transport system will be cloned and characterized.

Regulation of Proximal P_i Reabsorption

Phosphate balance of intake and output is largely controlled by a variety of hormonal and nonhormonal factors which regulate renal (proximal tubular) P_i reabsorption; predominant examples are parathyroid hormone (PTH), growth factors and dietary phosphate intake [for a complete discussion of the regulation of renal P_i handling the reader is referred to several recent reviews, e.g. 1–4, 6, 22]. Since the apical Na/P_i cotransport represents a rate-limiting step for proximal P_i reabsorption (see above), this transport system would be an ideal target for regulation. In fact most of the known physiologically important modulators of renal P_i reabsorption have been shown to alter the rate of apical Na/P_i cotransport.

Currently we are aware of the following three possibilities of how the apical P_i entry step (Na/P_i cotransport) can be regulated immediately, that is within hours [for discussion of long-term effects, see 6, 23].

Allosteric Regulation. Allosteric regulation of Na/P_i cotransport is mostly related to changes of the concentration of protons at either the cytoplasmic or luminal membrane surface and seems to be a direct consequence of the kinetic properties of the Na/P_i cotransport system [24]. As demonstrated with isolated brush-border membrane vesicles the rate of Na/P_i cotransport is highly dependent on the external pH value: transport is roughly doubled when the pH value increases from 7 to 8 [25]. Alterations of renal P_i reabsorption as observed in acute changes of the acid-base status or changes due to an altered metabolic activity (e.g. gluconeogenesis) might therefore be explained by an allosteric regulation by protons of the apical Na/P_i cotransport.

Protein Synthesis-Independent Regulation. In principle this kind of regulation could be achieved by either posttranslational modification(s) of the transporter molecule itself or by regulatory protein(s). Alternatively protein synthesis-independent regulation might also involve a recruitment of silent/inactive transport units or a retrieval of transporters by endocytic/exocytic mechanisms to alter rapidly the number of transport units within the membrane [6].

With brush-border membranes isolated from rat kidney and established renal epithelial cell lines (mainly OK cells) a large body of evidence was obtained that parathyroid hormone regulates (inhibits) apical Na/P_i cotransport by a decrease of the maximal transport rate V_{max}; in OK cells no inhibition of the basolaterally localized Na/P_i transport has been observed [26]. Recent evidence has indicated that PTH activates both adenyl cyclase (leading to an activation of protein kinase A via elevated cAMP) and phospholipase C. Activation of the later subsequently leads to an increased intracellular level of diacylglycerol and inositol triphosphate, both products being involved in activation of protein kinase C [6, 22, 27].

A direct relationship between the two intracellular signalling cascades (protein kinase A/C) and the inactivation of the Na/P_i cotransport system by PTH has not yet been determined at a molecular level. The participation of the protein kinase activities A and/or C in PTH action however suggests that phosphorylation reactions represent a key event in the inhibition of Na/P_i cotransport; yet a direct phosphorylation of Na/P_i transport systems remains to be demonstrated. Since there is also evidence for an endocytic retrieval of Na/P_i transport systems upon PTH action, phosphorylation of regulatory protein(s) eventually being involved cannot be excluded [6, 7].

Protein Synthesis-Dependent Regulation. In general most in vivo maneuvers which stimulate proximal tubular P_i reabsorption, so that the effect is retained at the level of isolated membranes, increase the rate of apical Na/P_i transport (manifested by an increase of V_{max}) in a protein synthesis-dependent manner. On the basis of isolated brush-border membranes and cultured renal cells evidence for a protein synthesis-dependent increase of apical Na/P_i transport was obtained for the effect of growth hormones and insulin-like growth factors, thyroid hormone and (most thoroughly investigated) for the situation of P_i deprivation (P_i diet, adaption) [6, 22, 23]. Interestingly, inhibition of Na/P_i transport as observed after multiple injections of glucocorticoids is also dependent on protein synthesis [28].

The mammalian kidney responds to a low P_i diet with increased renal (proximal tubular) P_i reabsorption which is expressed in an increased rate of apical Na/P_i cotransport. To a large part this adaptive response is independent of the hormonal status of the organism and thus represents an intrinsic adaptive phenomenon of the proximal epithelial cell [1, 3, 29, 30]. P_i transport studies with brush-border membranes isolated from rats fed a low P_i diet and which were additionally treated with actinomycin D suggested that under P_i deprivation conditions Na/P_i cotransport is under control of protein de novo synthesis and/or of altered transcription [31]. Regulation of Na/P_i cotransport by changes of the extracellular concentration of P_i has since been mimicked with a variety of established renal cell lines [6]. The use of different drugs to inhibit translation clearly indicated that the adaptive increase of Na/P_i cotransport is strictly dependent on protein de novo synthesis. Interestingly, the adaptive increase of Na/P_i cotransport could also be blocked by cordycepin (3′-deoxyadenosine), which presumably inhibits polyadenylation and thus interferes with the synthesis of mRNA. To further investigate the interesting possibility of a posttranscriptional but pretranslational control mechanism, knowledge about the nature of the protein(s) and mRNA(s) involved would be needed.

In the context of protein synthesis-dependent regulation of Na/P_i cotransport it should also be mentioned that different groups have reported an apparent correlation between increased Na/P_i cotransport (due to P_i restriction) and membrane fluidity [32, 33]. The influence of the lipid composition of the membrane on the rate of Na/P_i cotransport, however, is still not known and would require detailed knowledge of the nature of the Na/P_i transport protein.

Identification of Na/P_i Cotransport Systems

Our current view of the regulatory mechanisms controlling renal P_i reabsorption via modulation of proximal tubular apical Na/P_i cotransport is mainly derived from studies using whole cells (cell cultures) and isolated brush-border membrane vesicles and thus remains partly hypothetical until the molecular identity of (the) apical Na/P_i cotransport system(s) is known. We briefly discuss first attempts made to identify apical Na/P_i cotransport systems and then expose current progress made with regard to the molecular cloning of renal Na/P_i cotransporters.

Biochemical Approaches

Within the last 10 years various groups have tried to identify apical Na/P_i cotransport systems on the basis of covalent labeling and reconstitution techniques. This approach turned out to be rather difficult mainly because no specific inhibitor of the Na/P_i cotransport system with high affinity is currently known. One exception might be a derivative of phosphonoformic acid which competitively inhibits Na/P_i cotransport [34]. Thus, due to the different methods used the picture emerging from these attempts is rather complex and has not led to an unequivocal identification of the Na/P_i cotransport system. Purification and reconstitution experiments provided some evidence for a hydrophobic peptide of low molecular weight (phosphorin) for which P_i binding has been demonstrated [35]. Since however P_i binding was not Na-dependent, involvement of this peptide in Na/P_i cotransport remains questionable. In similar experiments a protein of approximately 70 kDa was described exhibiting P_i binding [36]. Very recently the same authors reported the purification of an approximately 64-kDa protein from rabbit kidney brush-border membranes [37]. Reconstitution of the purified protein fraction into liposomes demonstrated Na-dependent uptake of P_i. A possible identity of this protein which can be extracted by organic solvents to a recently cloned Na/P_i cotransport protein from rabbit kidney (see below) remains to be demonstrated.

Although several reports pointed to a functional importance of certain amino acid residues such as arginine residues (inhibition of P_i transport by phenylglyoxal [38] or SH groups [39]), the use of functionally important amino acid residues for a structural identification by covalent labeling techniques has been reported in only one study. Based on the observation that acetylimidazole was capable of inhibiting P_i transport in OK cells in a P_i-protectable manner proteins of a M_r of 31, 53 and 105 kDa have been described as possible candidates for the Na/P_i cotransport system in these cells [40]. Recently, using azido-NAD, two proteins of M_r of 70 and 97 kDa were identified in rat brush-border membranes [41]. None of the mentioned proteins have been further characterized, such as by amino acid sequencing, and therefore remain potential candidates for a renal Na/P_i transport system.

Target size analysis performed with isolated rat kidney cortex brush-border membranes resulted in a functional molecular mass of apical Na/P_i cotransport of around 240 kDa [42]. Assuming a molecular weight of between 50 and 100 kDa (see also below), these results could indicate that the functional apical Na/P_i cotransport system could be of a (hetero- or homo-) oligomeric structure.

Molecular Cloning of Renal Na/P_i Cotransport Systems

Cloning of a Na/P_i Transport System from Rabbit Kidney Cortex. Since the first successful molecular cloning of a membrane transport system with the use of oocytes of the clawed frog *Xenopus laevis* as expression system (cloning by expression [43]) this method has been successfully used to clone and identify a variety of membrane transport systems. Using this cloning strategy we recently described the molecular cloning of a first Na-dependent P_i transport system (from rabbit cortex, referred to as NaPi-1 [44]).

After the first observations made, namely that injection of poly(A)$^+$RNA isolated from rabbit kidney cortex into oocytes lead to an expression of Na/P_i cotransport additionally to the intrinsic Na/P_i transport activity and that most likely one polypeptide chain is involved in this expression (evidence obtained by size fractionation of mRNA [45]), a cDNA library was set up. By screening the library a single clone with an insert of an approximate length of 1.8 kB was identified [44]. Importantly, the apparent K_m values for the interaction with P_i and Na as observed after injection of the cloned cRNA were similar as the K_m values described with rabbit brush-border membranes. Of special interest was the observation that the apparent K_m value for the interaction with Na of expressed activity (50–60 m*M*) was different compared to the corresponding value found in water injected oocytes (10–20 m*M*) since this observation indicated that increased transport activity due to injection of cloned cRNA might indeed represent a true expression of injected cRNA rather than a possible activation of intrinsic Na/P_i transport activity.

The open reading frame of the cloned NaPi-1 cDNA predicts a primary peptide structure of 465 amino acids (calculated molecular mass of 51,797). The molecular weight of the major product observed after in vitro translation of NaPi-1 cRNA in the absence of microsomes was determined as 41 kDa (see fig. 2). In the presence of microsomes this 41-kDa form is shifted partially to a 49-kDa form due to glycosylation; treatment with endoglucosidase-H reverted the 49-kDa form back to the 41-kDa form [data not shown]. Hydrophobicity analysis of the primary NaPi-1 amino acid sequence predicts a membrane protein exhibiting 6–8 transmembrane-spanning domains. Assuming that all of the four potential N-glycosylation sites are glycosylated, both the N and C termini would be localized at the cytoplasmic membrane surface; the precise molecular arrangement of NaPi-1 within the membrane, however, is currently not yet known.

Using NaPi-1-derived probes strong hybridization was observed in Northern blots with mRNA isolated from rabbit kidney cortex and to a weaker extent also with mRNA isolated from rabbit liver [44]; the precise localization of NaPi-1 mRNA in the liver is not known at present. Notably, no hybridization signal was detected with mRNA isolated from small intestinal mucosa. These observations suggest that the cloned Na/P_i transport system NaPi-1 does not represent a ubiquitous transport system; e.g. it cannot be regarded as a 'housekeeping' Na/P_i transport activity as present in every cell membrane.

To localize the cloned Na/P_i cotransport system both at the protein and mRNA level, an antibody against a synthetic peptide [14-mer derived from the C terminus) has been

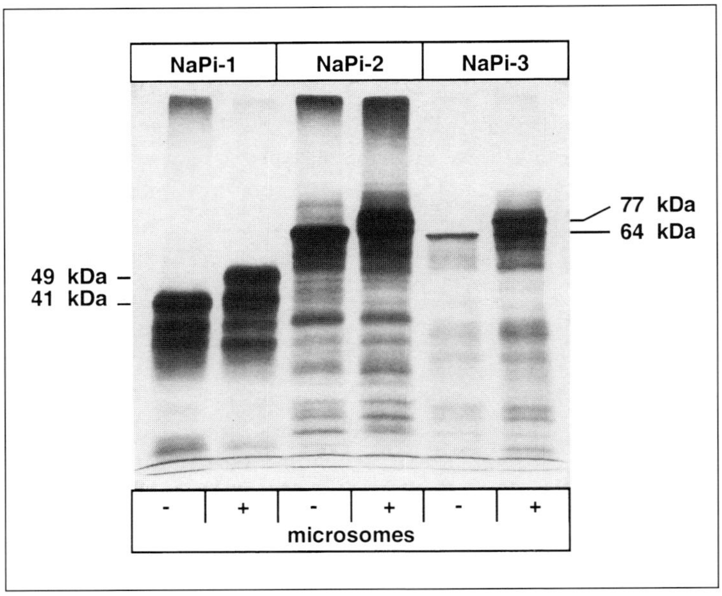

Fig. 2. In vitro translations of cloned renal Na/P_i cotransporter cRNAs. In vitro transcribed cRNAs of the Na/P_i cotransporter clones NaPi-1 (rabbit), NaPi-2 (rat) and NaPi-3 (human) were used for in vitro translation in the absence (−) or presence (+) of pancreatic microsomes [for details, see 44].

raised and polychain reaction after reverse transcription (RT-PCR) has been applied in microdissected nephron segments. In Western blots using brush-border membranes isolated from rabbit kidney cortex, a protein with a M_r of approximately 60–64 kDa was recognized by the antibody obtained. This reaction with a 60/64-kDa protein would be consistent with the NaPi-1 protein being glycosylated at 3–4 of the potential N-glycosylation sites (assuming approximately 4 kDa per glycosylation site). On the basis of the Western blot technique the reaction with the 60/64-kDa protein could be attributed to the apical membrane since after a separation of brush-border and basolateral membranes by free-flow electrophoresis the 60/64-kDa protein was found to migrate parallel to the apical membrane marker enzyme leucine-aminopeptidase [46].

This anti-(NaPi-1) antibody has been further used in immunofluorescence studies to localize the NaPi-1 related protein in rabbit kidney cortex. These studies demonstrated anti-(NaPi-1)-antibody-mediated fluorescence exclusively in the apical membrane of proximal tubular cells; no distinction between the functionally different proximal tubular segments S_1, S_2 and S_3 could be made on the basis of immunofluorescence [unpubl. data].

The localization of NaPi-1 as suggested by the immunofluorescence studies could be confirmed by RT-PCR experiments using microdissected nephron segments of the rabbit kidney. Using specific oligonucleotide primers for NaPi-1, the corresponding mRNA was found in proximal tubules only [S_1, S_2 and S_3 segments of both superficial and deep nephrons; unpubl. data]. As already indicated by immunofluorescence, no NaPi-1-specific mRNA could be detected by RT-PCR in other nephron segments such as in the loop of Henle and in the distal and collecting ducts. These studies clearly indicate that the Na/P_i cotransport system NaPi-1 represents (at least) one of the Na/P_i cotransport systems of the apical membrane of rabbit proximal tubules. The exact functional role of NaPi-1 (e.g. as a target for regulation) remains to be clarified. Additionally, the possibility of the existence of various isoforms of Na/P_i cotransport systems in the proximal tubule of the rabbit kidney remains to be investigated.

Molecular Cloning of Rat and Human Kidney Cortex Na/P_i Cotransport Systems. Northern blots using NaPi-1-specific probes and mRNAs isolated from kidney cortex of various species indicated that NaPi-1 shows poor or no homology to renal Na/P_i transport systems of other species. This finding led us to clone by expression a Na/P_i cotransport system of the rat and human kidney cortex. Starting from mRNA isolated from the respective kidney cortex, we were recently able to isolate a clone coding for a rat (NaPi-2) and a human (NaPi-3) Na/P_i transport system. Analysis of expressed Na/P_i transport after injection of NaPi-2 or NaPi-3 cRNA into oocytes demonstrated sigmoidal dependence of the concentration of Na ions (Hill coefficient of around two) and pH dependence similar to that observed in rat kidney brush-border membranes.

The primary structures of the encoded proteins NaPi-2 and NaPi-3 are not yet known. Evidence that the newly cloned Na/P_i transport systems NaPi-2 and NaPi-3 might belong to a different group of renal Na/P_i transport proteins than NaPi-1 was obtained by the following observations: (1) in vitro translation (in the absence or presence of microsomes) of NaPi-2 and NaPi-3 cRNAs resulted in products of similar molecular weights but different compared to the in vitro translation products of NaPi-1 cRNA (fig. 2), and (2) Northern blot experiments indicated that NaPi-2 and NaPi-3 hybridize to each other but not to NaPi-1 [data not shown].

Similarity to Other Na-Dependent Cotransporters. So far no sequence homology of NaPi-1 (a rabbit kidney cortex Na/P_i transporter) was found within current data banks. Notably, there seems to be no homolgy to the SGLT1 family (small intestinal Na/glucose transporter family) nor to the GAT-1 family (derived from the rat brain Na/Cl/GABA cotransporter) [47]. However, one structural motif, the SOB motif (Gly-X-X-X-X-Leu-X-X-X-Gly-Arg, where x is any amino acid) seems to be conserved in NaPi-1, with the exception of the replacement of a proline for the second glycine. The functional significance of this motif has been suggested to be related to the sodium binding site [48], though it has not yet been established. This partial similarity to other cloned Na/solute transport systems might implicate that the cloned Na/Na/P_i transport system NaPi-1 might belong to a larger family of Na-dependent cotransport systems despite the lack of overall sequence homology. At present no information about similar motifs or possible homologies to other Na-solute transport systems of the newly cloned Na/P_i cotransporters NaPi-2 and NaPi-3 is available.

Conclusions

As outlined in the first part, proximal tubular apical Na/P_i transport represents a main target for the regulation of renal P_i reabsorption. The central role of this membrane transport process and the most likely mechanisms of its regulation have emerged from functional (transport) studies mainly using isolated membranes and established cell cultures. With the recently obtained knowledge on the molecular identity of some renal Na/P_i cotransport systems, it is now possible to elucidate the mechanisms of the regulation of renal P_i reabsorption at a molecular level. Using the newly available molecular tools, such as antibodies and oligonucleotide probes, work in progress concentrates on the precise localization of Na/P_i transport systems within the nephron and on the regulatory control mechanisms of the individual transport systems. With regard to protein synthesis-independent and -dependent regulatory mechanisms of Na/P_i cotransport it will be of interest to analyze for possible posttranslational modifications (e.g. phosphorylation upon PTH action) and to clarify the postulated regulation of Na/P_i cotransport, for example by an altered rate of transcription and/or stability of the corresponding mRNA. Furthermore, studies on the molecular structure/function relationships will eventually lead to an understanding of the transport mechanisms and clarify the role of Na ions and protons (see allosteric regulation) on a molecular basis.

To answer unequivocally the many questions raised, attention should again be drawn to the likely existence of several isoforms of apical Na/P_i cotransport systems which possibly might play different roles in the regulatory control of P_i reabsorption. With the help of the recently cloned Na/P_i transport systems NaPi-1 (rabbit), NaPi-2 (rat) and NaPi-3 (human) it will eventually be possible to identify additional isoforms of proximal tubular apical Na/P_i cotransport systems.

Acknowledgement

Work performed in the authors' laboratory was generously supported by the Swiss National Fonds (grants No. 32-28664.90 to J. B. and No. 32-30785.91 to H. M.).

References

1 Berndt TJ, Kmox FG: Renal regulation of phosphate excretion; in Seldin GW, Giebisch G (eds): The Kidney, Physiology and Pathophysiology. New York, Raven Press, 1992, pp 2511–2532.
2 Mizgala CL, Quamme GA: Renal handling of phosphate. Physiol Rev 1985;65:431–466.
3 Bonjour J-P, Caverzasio J: Phosphate transport in the kidney. Rev Physiol Biochem Pharmacol 1984; 100:161–214.
4 Murer H, Biber J: Renal tubular phosphate transport; in Seldin DW, Giebisch G (eds): The Kidney, Physiology and Pathophysiology. New York, Raven Press, 1992, pp 2481–2509.
5 Hammerman MR: Phosphate transport across renal proximal tubular cell membranes. Am J Physiol 1986;251:F385–F398.
6 Murer H, Werner A, Reshkin S, Wuarin F, Biber J: Cellular mechanisms in proximal tubular reabsorption of inorganic phosphate. Am J Physiol 1991;260:C885–C899.
7 Biber J: Cellular aspects of proximal tubular phosphate reabsorption. Kidney Int 1989;36:360–369.
8 Dennis VW, Woodhall PB, Robinson RR: Characteristics of phosphate transport in isolated proximal tubule. Am J Physiol 1976;231:979–985.
9 Baumann K, De Rouffignac C, Roinel N, Rumrich G, Ullrich KJ: Renal phosphate transport: Inhomogeneity of local proximal transport rates and sodium dependence. Pflügers Arch 1975;356:287–297.
10 Hoffman N, Thees M, Kinne R: Phosphate transport by isolated renal brush border vesicles. Pflügers Arch 1976;362:147–156.
11 Beliveau R, Strevey J: Kinetic model for phosphate transport in renal brush border membranes. Am J Physiol 1988;254:F329–F336.
12 Frömter E: Viewing the kidney through microelectrodes. Am J Physiol 1984;247:F695–F705.
13 Freeman D, Bartlett S, Radda G, Ross B: Energetics of sodium transport in the kidney: Saturation transfer ^{31}P-NMR. Biochim Biophys Acta 1983;762:325–336.
14 Hagenbuch B, Murer H: Phosphate transport across the basolateral membrane from the rat kidney cortex: Sodium dependence? Pflügers Arch 1986;407:S149–S155.
15 Ullrich K, Papavassiliou F, Rumrich G, Fritsch G: Contraluminal phosphate transport in the proximal tubule of rat kidney. Pflügers Arch 1985;405:106–109.
16 Schwab SJ, Kahr S, Hammerman MR: Na-gradient dependent P_i uptake in basolateral membrane vesicles from dog kidney. Am J Physiol 1984;246:F663–F669.

17 Reshkin SJ, Forgo J, Murer H: Functional asymmetry of phosphate transport and its regulation in OK-cells: Phosphate transport. Pfügers Arch 1990;416:554–560.

18 Walker JJ, Yan TS, Quamme GA: Presence of multiple sodium-dependent phosphate transport processes in proximal brush-border membranes. Am J Physiol 1987; 252:F226–F231.

19 Brunette MG, Chan M, Maag U, Beliveau R: Phosphate uptake by superficial and deep nephron brush border membranes. Effect of dietary phosphate and parathyroid hormone. Pfügers Arch 1984;400: 356–362.

20 Quamme GA: Effect of pH on Na-dependent phosphate transport in renal outer cortical and outer medullary BBMV. Am J Physiol 1990; 258:F1–F8.

21 Levi M: Heterogeneity of Pi transport by BBMV from superficial and juxtamedullary cortex of rat. Am J Physiol 1990;258:F1616–F1624.

22 Hammerman MR: The growth hormone-insulin-like growth factor axis in the kidney. Am J Physiol 1989; 257:F503–F514.

23 Murer H: Cellular mechanisms in proximal tubular Pi reabsorption: Some answers and many more questions. J Am Soc Nephrol 1992; 2:1649–1665.

24 Gmaj P, Murer H: Cellular mechanisms of inorganic phosphate transport in kidney. Physiol Rev 1986;66: 36–70.

25 Amstutz M, Mohrmann M, Gmaj P, Murer H: Effect of pH on phosphate transport in rat renal brush border membrane vesicles. Am J Physiol 1985;248:F705–F710.

26 Reshkin SJ, Forgo J, Murer H: Functional asymmetry in phosphate transport and its regulation in OK-cells: Parathyroid hormone hormone inhibition. Pfügers Arch 1990;416:624–631.

27 Hruska KA, Moskowitz D, Esprit P, Citivelli R, Westbrook S, Huskey M: Stimulation of inositol triphosphate and diacylglycerol production in renal tubular cells by parathyroid hormone. J Clin Invest 1987;79:230–239.

28 Freiberg JM, Kinsella J, Sacktor B: Glucocorticoids increase the Na–H exchange and decrease the Na-gradient dependent phosphate uptake systems in renal brush border membranes vesicles. Proc Natl Acad Sci USA 1982;79:4932–4936.

29 Knochel JP: The clinical physiological implications of phosphorus deficiency; in Seldin GW, Giebisch G (eds): The Kidney, Physiology and Pathophysiology. New York, Raven Press, 1992, pp 2533–2562.

30 Escoubet B, Djabali K, Amiel C: Adaption to Pi deprivation of the cell Na-dependent Pi uptake: A widespread process. Am J Physiol 1989;256:C322–C328.

31 Shah SV, Kempson SA, Northrup TE, Dousa TP: Renal adaption to a low phosphate diet in rats: Blockade by actinomycin D. J Clin Invest 1979;64:955–966.

32 Levi M, Baird BM, Wilson PV: Cholesterol modulates rat renal brush border membranes phosphate transport. J Clin Invest 1990; 85:231–237.

33 Molitoris BA, Alfrey AC, Harris RA, Simon FR: Renal apical membrane cholesterol and fluidity in regulation of phosphate transport. Am J Physiol 1985;249:F12–F19.

34 Hoppe A, Lin J-T, Onsgard M, Knox FG, Dousa TP: Quantitation of the Na-Pi cotransporter in renal cortical brush border membranes. J Biol Chem 1991;266:11528–11536.

35 Kessler RJ, Vaughn DA, Fanestil DD: Identifaction of a phosphate binding proteolipid from brush border. J Biol Chem 1982;257:14311–14317.

36 Debiec H, Lorenc R: Identification of Na,P_i-binding protein in kidney and intestinal brush border membranes. Biochem J 1988;255:185–191.

37 Debiec H, Lorenc R, Ronco PM: Reconstitution and characterization of a Na/P_i-cotransporter protein from rabbit kidney brush border membranes. Biochem J 1992;286: 97–102.

38 Strevey J, Vachon V, Beaumier B, Giroux S, Beliveau R: Characterization of essential arginine residues implicated in the renal transport of phosphate and glucose. Biochim Biophys Acta 1992;1106:110–116.

39 Loghman Adham M: Characterization of essential sulfhydryl groups of rat renal Na-Pi cotransporter. Am J Physiol 1991;260:F874–F882.

40 Wuarrin F, Wu K, Murer H, Biber J: The Na/P_i-cotransporter of OK-cell: Reaction and tentative identification with N-acetylimidazole. Biochim Biophys Acta 1989;981:185–192.

41 Al-Mahrouq MA, Kempson SA: Photoaffinity labeling of brush-border membrane proteins which bind phosphonoformic acid. J Biol Chem 1991;266:1422–1427.

42 Beliveau R, Demeule M, Ibnoul-Khatib H, Bergeron M, Beauregard G, Potier M: Radiation-inactivation studies on brush border membrane vesicles. General considerations and application to the glucose and phosphate carriers. Biochem J 1988;252:807–813.

43 Hediger MA, Coaday MJ, Ikeda TS, Wright EM: Expression cloning and cDNA sequencing of the Na/glucose cotransporter. Nature 1987; 330:379–381.

44 Werner A, Moore ML, Mantei N, Biber J, Semenza G, Murer H: Cloning and expression of cDNA for a Na/Pi cotransport system of kidney cortex. Proc Natl Acad Sci USA 1991;88:9608–9612.

45 Werner A, Biber J, Forgo J, Palacin M, Murer H: Expression or renal transport systems for inorganic phosphate and sulphate in *Xenopus laevis* oocytes. J Biol Chem 1990; 265:12331–12336.

46 Biber J, Werner A, Moore M, Murer H: Polyclonal antibodies against the renal Na/Pi-cotransporter. J Am Soc Nephrol 1991;2:616.

47 Wright EM, Hager KM, Turk E: Sodium cotransport proteins. Curr Opin Cell Biol 1992;4:696–702.

48 Deguchi Y, Yamato I, Ankraku Y: Nucleotide sequence of qlts, the Na/glutamate symport carrier gene of *Escherichia coli* B. J Biol Chem 1990;265:21704–21708.

Original Paper

Renal Physiol Biochem 1993;16:48–65

The Biological Significance of Cell Volume

F. Lang[a]
M. Ritter[a]
H. Völkl[a]
D. Häussinger[b]

[a] Institute for Physiology, University of Innsbruck, Austria;
[b] Department for Internal Medicine, University of Freiburg, FRG

Abstract

To survive, cells have to avoid excessive alterations of their volume. To this end, cells have developed a complex machinery of cell volume regulatory mechanisms comprising transport across the cell membrane and metabolism. Upon cell swelling, they loose electrolytes mainly via selective K^+ channels and unselective ion channels and/or KCl symport, upon cell shrinkage they accumulate ions by Na^+,K^+,$2Cl^-$ cotransport and parallel operation of Na^+/H^+ exchange and Cl^-/HCO_3^- exchange. In addition, cell shrinkage stimulates glycogenolysis, proteolysis and formation of organic osmolytes such as amino acids, methylamines and polyols. Cell swelling stimulates formation of glycogen and proteins and cellular release of organic osmolytes. Alterations of cell volume do play a crucial role in the regulation of cell function, as illustrated by four examples:

1. Epithelial transport may lead to cell swelling, which then triggers volume regulatory mechanisms modifying transcellular transport.

2. Insulin swells hepatocytes by activation of Na^+,K^+,$2Cl^-$ cotransport and Na^+/H^+ exchange, glucagon shrinks those cells by activation of ion channels. The respective volume changes participate in the regulation of cellular protein and glycogen metabolism by these hormones.

3. Growth factors and expression of ras oncogene activate Na^+,K^+,$2Cl^-$ cotransport and Na^+/H^+ exchange, leading to the respective cell swelling.

4. Hepatocyte swelling triggers a hepatorenal reflex decreasing renal blood flow.

Key Words

Liver
Kidney
Insulin
Glucagon
Na^+/H^+ Exchange
Na^+, K^+, $2Cl^-$ Cotransport
Ion channels
Proteolysis
Ras Oncogene

Prof. Dr. F. Lang
Institute for Physiology
University of Innsbruck
Fritz-Pregl-Strasse 3
A-6010 Innsbruck (Austria)

1011–6524/93/
0162–0048 $2.75/0

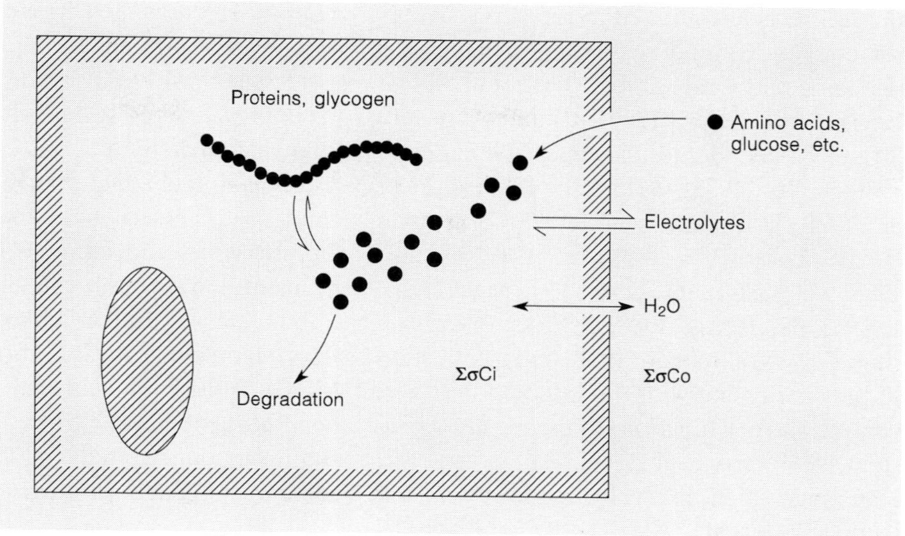

Fig. 1. Factors compromising the constancy of cell volume. The osmotic equilibrium across the cell membrane is achieved, when $\Sigma\ \sigma \times c_i \approx \Sigma\ \sigma \times c_o$, where σ is the reflection coefficient, c_i the intra- and c_o the extracellular concentration of each particular solvent. It is challenged by transport of osmotically active substances (such as glucose, amino acids or electrolytes) across the cell membrane, as well as by cellular metabolism, such as degradation of glucose and amino acids, formation or degradation of macromolecules (such as glycogen, proteins), which are osmotically less active than the sum of their monomers.

Introduction

To survive, cells have to avoid excessive swelling or shrinkage. With few exceptions, the cell membranes of mammalian cells are highly permeable to water and too fragile to resist significant hydrostatic pressure gradients. Thus, to preserve their volume cells have to create an osmotic equilibrium across the cell membrane [Lang et al., 1990]. Accordingly, the sum of the osmotically active substances must be approximately equal in intra- and extracellular fluid (fig. 1).

The osmotic equilibrium is, however, permanently compromised by alterations of extracellular osmolarity and, more importantly, by cellular transport and metabolism of osmotically active substances (fig. 1).

Thus, during the course of evolution cells had to learn strategies to regulate their volume. Those strategies are probably among the best preserved cellular functions.

In the past decades, a multitude of cell volume regulatory mechanisms has been disclosed, operating in a wide variety of cells. However, it has been only recently that the significance of cell volume and cell volume regulatory mechanisms has been recognized for the function of cells, organs and organisms. As a matter of fact, the volume regulatory mechanisms comprise a complex machinery, participating in the regulation of cellular function. This machinery can be turned on and off during transport and metabolism and by hormones and mediators.

In the following volume regulatory mechanisms and examples of their participation in cellular function will be presented. The paper will concentrate on observations made in the authors' laboratories. For further information the reader is encouraged to refer to previous reviews on volume regulatory mechanisms [Ballanyi and Grafe, 1988; Beck et al., 1988; Beck and Guder, 1989; Chamberlin and Strange, 1989; Deutsch and Lee, 1988; Geck, 1989; Gilles, 1988; Goldstein, 1989; Graf et al., 1988; Hoffmann et al., 1988; Hoffmann and Simonsen, 1989; Kleinzeller, 1989; Lauf, 1988; Macknight and Leaf, 1977; Macknight, 1987, 1988; Reuss, 1988; Schultz, 1989; Ussing, 1989; Völkl, et al., 1988] and a collection of papers dealing with the interaction of cell volume and cell function [Bianchini and Grinstein, 1992; Graf et al., 1992; Halestrap, 1992; Häussinger et al., 1992; Hoffmann et al., 1992; Kimelberg et al., 1992; Kurtz and Scholz, 1992; Lang et al., 1992b; O'Neill, 1992].

Volume Regulatory Mechanisms

Upon cell swelling most cells release cellular electrolytes. The resulting decrease of intracellular osmolarity achieves a regulatory cell volume decrease (RVD). Cell shrinkage, on the other hand, triggers the uptake of electrocytes into the cells, leading to regulatory cell volume increase (RVI). In addition to electrolyte transport, cellular osmolarity is modified by transport of organic substances and metabolic formation or disposal of osmotically active subsances, contributing to RVD and RVI, respectively.

Volume Regulatory Electrolyte Loss

The various mechanisms reported to accomplish cellular electrolyte loss during RVD are listed in table 1. In most cells, cell swelling leads to the activation of K^+ channels and anion channels. The properties of volume regulatory ion channels in cultured Madin-Darby canine kidney (MDCK) cells are illustrated in figure 2. The K^+ channel is highly K^+ selective and slightly inwardly rectifying, i.e. depolarization decreases the single channel conductance [Weiss and Lang, 1992]. The K^+ channel is calcium-sensitive and upon cell swelling it is probably activated by an increase of intracellular calcium activity.

The anion channel poorly selects between chloride and bicarbonate and probably other anions [Weiss and Lang, 1992]. The mechanisms of activation of the anion channel are rather eclusive. In Ehrlich ascites tumor cells [Hoffmann et al., 1992; Lambert, 1987] and in MDCK cells [Paulmichl et al., 1989] but not in hepatocytes [Vom Dahl et al., 1991] circumstantial evidence points to the involvement of some lipoxygenase product.

Volume Regulatory Electrolyte Uptake

The cellular uptake of electrolytes during RVI is accomplished by the $Na^+,K^+,2Cl^-$ cotransporter and by the parallel operation of the Na^+/H^+ antiporter and the Cl^-/HCO_3^- antiporter (fig. 3, table 1). Simultaneously, in MDCK cells cellular electrolyte loss is minimized by inactivation of chloride channels and to a lesser extent of K^+ channels [Ritter et al., 1991b]. The activation of the Na^+/H^+ antiporter apparently surpasses the activation of the Cl^-/HCO_3^- antiporter, leading to intracellular alkalinization during cell shrinkage. The bulk of H^+ and HCO_3^- exchanged for Na^+ and Cl^-, respectively, is, however, replenished within the cell from CO_2. Thus, the net effect of the Na^+/H^+ exchange and Cl^-/HCO_3^- exchange is cellular gain of NaCl. Sodium entering the cell via the $Na^+,K^+,2Cl^-$ cotransport or via the Na^+/H^+ antiport is rapidly exchanged for K^+ by the Na^+/K^+ ATPase. Thus, the ion transporters eventually serve to accumulate cellular KCl.

The ion channels inactivated by cell shrinkage appear to be distinct from the ion channels activated during cell swelling, which are virtually closed at isovolumetric conditions [Ritter et al., 1991b].

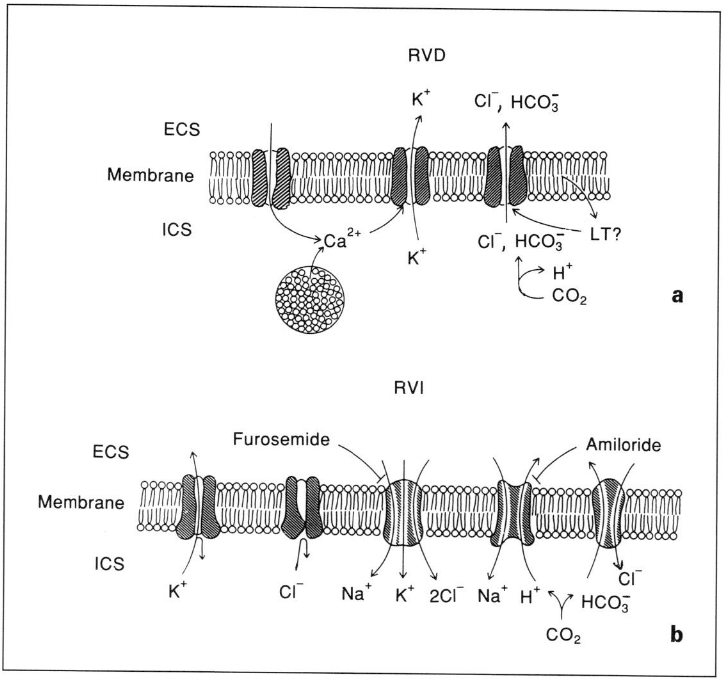

Fig. 2. Volume regulatory ion transport. **a** Cell swelling activates selective K^+ channels and unselective anion channels. The cellular loss of electrolytes reduces the intracellular osmolarity and thus allows RVD. The K^+ channels are activated by intracellular calcium, which comes from intracellular fluid and/or intracellular stores. Activation of anion channels may involve leukotrienes (LT). **b** Cell shrinkage leads to activation of the $Na^+,K^+,2Cl^-$ cotransporter and the parallel activation of the Na^+/H^+ antiporter and the Cl^-/HCO_3^- antiporter. The cellular accumulation of electrolytes via these carriers allows RVI. Simultaneously K^+ and Cl^- channels are closed to reduce cellular loss of electrolytes. ECS = Extracellular space; ICS = intracellular space.

The mechanisms accounting for the activation of $Na^+,K^+,2Cl^-$ cotransport and of Na^+/H^+ antiport as well as for the inactivation of the ion channels are poorly understood. Both, the $Na^+,K^+,2Cl^-$ cotransporter and the Na^+/H^+ antiporter are modified by phosphorylation and both are most likely attached to the cytoskeleton [Bianchini and Grinstein, 1992; Sardet et al., 1990, 1991]. It could be speculated that alterations of cell volume may be sensed by the cytoskeleton, and that the phosphorylation site serves to modify the sensitivity or the respective carrier to alterations of cell volume.

Transport and Metabolism of Nonelectrolytes

As listed in table 1, alterations of cell volume modify the transport and metabolism of amino acids, polyols (such as sorbitol and inositol) and methylamines (such as betaine and glycerophosphorylcholine). Cellular formation and accumulation of these osmolytes are stimulated by cell shrinkage, their release is stimulated by cell swelling. Furthermore, cell shrinkage activates the degradation of proteins to amino acids and of glycogen to glucosephosphate and their metabolites (table 1, fig. 1). The respective alterations of cellular osmolarity expectedly contribute to cell volume regulation. Other metabolic pathways, such as urea formation [Häussinger and Lang, 1990], are probably indirectly affected (fig. 4).

Table 1. Cell volume regulatory mechanisms

Mechanism	Cells/tissues [references]
Regulatory cell volume decrease	
Parallel activation of K^+ and Cl^- channels	Ehrlich ascites tumor cells [Hoffmann et al., 1984, 1986, 1988; Hoffmann, 1985a, b, 1987; Hudson and Schultz, 1988; Lang et al., 1987] Lymphocytes [Cheung et al., 1982; Deutsch and Lee, 1988; Grinstein et al., 1982a–c, 1983a, 1984; Sarkadi et al., 1984a, b, 1985] Platelets [Livne et al., 1987] Endothelial cells [O'Neill, 1992] Fibroblasts [Rugolo et al., 1989] Astrocytes [Kimelberg and Kettenmann, 1990; Kimelberg et al., 1990b, 1992] Choroid plexus [Christensen, 1987; Christensen et al., 1989] Ciliary epithelium [Farahbahksh and Fain, 1987; Yantorno et al., 1989] Eye lens [Beebe et al., 1990] Intestine [Germann et al., 1986; Hazama and Okada, 1988; Lau et al., 1984; MacLeod and Hamilton, 1990; Montero and Ilundain, 1989; Schultz et al., 1985; Wiener and Turnheim, 1990] MDCK cells [Paulmichl et al., 1989; Roy and Sauve 1987; Simons, 1984; Völkl et al., 1988] Frog skin [Costas et al., 1987; Ussing, 1986] Frog urinary bladder [Davis and Finn, 1985, 1987] Convoluted proximal renal tubules [Kirk et al., 1987a, 1987b; Sackin, 1987, 1989; Schild et al., 1991; Tauc et al., 1990; Welling et al., 1985; Welling and O'Neill, 1990] Liver [Häussinger et al., 1990c; Kristensen, 1986; Kristensen and Folke, 1984] Trachea [Butt et al., 1990; McCann et al., 1989]
Activation of electrogenic bicarbonate exit	Straight proximal renal tubules of the mouse kidney [Völkl and Lang, 1988a, b; Völkl et al., 1988] MDCK cells [Weiss and Lang, 1992]
Activation of KCl cotransport	Erythrocytes from toadfish [Lauf, 1982], birds [Kregenow, 1981], sheep [Dunham and Ellory, 1981; Ellory et al., 1985; Lauf, 1985] and man [O'Neill, 1987] Necturus gallbladder [Larson and Spring, 1984] Calcium-depleted Ehrlich ascites tumor cells [Kramhoft et al., 1986] Dog red cells with low intracellular sodium concentration [Parker, 1983a]
Activation of Na^+ entry	Frog skin [Costa et al., 1987] Urinary bladder [Finn and Reuss, 1975; Lewis et al., 1985]
Parallel operation of K^+/H^+ exchange and Cl^- HCO_3^- exchange	Amphiuma red cells [Cala, 1983; Cala et al., 1986] Frog skin [Ussing, 1990] Cornea [Bonanno, 1991]
K^+/H^+ ATPase	Gastric epithelium [Sernka, 1990]
Na^+/Ca^{2+} exchange and Ca^{2+}-ATPase	Dog red cells with high intracellular sodium concentration [Parker et al., 1975; Parker, 1978, 1979]
Loss of cellular amino acids [Bevan et al., 1990; Fincham et al., 1987; Fugelli and Rohrs, 1980; Hoffmann and Hendil, 1976; Hoffmann and Lambert, 1983; Kimelberg et al., 1990a, King and Goldstein, 1983; Law and Turner, 1987; Pasantes-Morales and Schousboe, 1988; Roy and Sauve, 1987; Sanchez Olea et al., 1991; Thurston et al., 1981, Vislie 1983]	
Loss of cellular polyoles [Garcia-Perez and Burg, 1990, 1991; Garty et al., 1991; Moriyama et al., 1990; Siebens and Spring, 1989; Yamauchi et al., 1991]	
Loss of cellular methylamines [Garcia-Perez and Burg, 1990, 1991; Garty et al., 1991; Moriyama et al., 1990; Siebens and Spring, 1989; Yamauchi et al., 1991]	
Net glycogen synthesis [Baquet et al., 1990; Lang et al., 1989]	
Net protein synthesis [Hallbrucker et al., 1991a; Häussinger et al., 1990a, b, 1991; Häussinger and Lang, 1991a, b]	

Table 1. (continued)

Regulatory cell volume increase

Parallel activation of Na^+/H^+ exchange and Cl^-/HCO_3^- exchange
- Amphiuma [Cala, 1980, 1983, 1985; Kregenow et al., 1985; Siebens and Kregenow 1985], rabbit [Jennings et al., 1986] and dog [Parker, 1983b; Parker and Castranova 1984] red cells
- Lymphocytes [Grinstein et al., 1983b, Grinstein et al., 1984, 1985a, b]
- Osteoclasts [Green et al., 1988]
- Endothelial cells [O'Neill and Klein, 1992]
- Parotis [Soltoff et al., 1989]
- Pancreas [Muallem and Loessberg, 1990]

- Gallbladder [Ericson and Spring, 1982; Fisher et al., 1981; Reuss, 1984; Spring 1985]
- Liver [Häussinger et al., 1990c]
- Medullary thick ascending limb of the kidney [Blumenfeld et al., 1989]
- Medullary collecting duct [Sun and Hebert, 1989]
- Proximal tubule [Lohr et al., 1989]
- MDCK cells [Ritter et al., 1991b]

NaCl-KCl symport or NaCl symport
- Avian [Bakker-Grunwald, 1981; Kregenow, 1981; Schmidt and McManus, 1977a–c], ferret [Mercer and Hoffmann, 1985], rat [Duhm and Göbel, 1984] and human [Adragna and Tosteson, 1984; O'Neill and Mikkelsen, 1987] red cells
- Ehrlich ascites tumor cells [Geck et al., 1980; Geck and Heinz, 1986; Hoffmann et al., 1983, 1988]
- 3T3 cells [Bakker-Grunwald et al., 1982]
- HeLa cells [Tivey et al., 1985]
- Frog skin [Ussing, 1985, 1986]
- Astrocytes [Kimelberg and Frangakis, 1986; Tas et al., 1987]
- Retinal pigment epithelium [Adorante and Miller, 1990]
- C6 glioma cells [Chassande et al., 1988]
- Intestine [MacLeod and Hamilton, 1990]
- Trachea [Musch and Field, 1989]
- Rabbit medullary thick ascending limb cells [Blumenfeld et al., 1989; Eveloff and Calamia, 1986]
- OK cells [Montrose et al., 1988]
- MDCK cells (Ritter et al., 1991b]
- Parotis [Soltoff et al., 1989]

Inhibition of K^+ and/or Cl^--channels
- MDCK cells [Ritter et al., 1991a]

- Frog skin [Costa et al., 1987; Leibowich et al., 1988]
- Urinary bladder [Donaldson et al., 1989; Lewis et al., 1985]
- Gallbladder [Stoddard and Reuss, 1989]
- Intestine [Montero and Ilundain, 1989]
- Proximal tubule [Lapointe et al., 1990]
- Heart cells [Drewnowska and Baumgarten, 1991; Frelin et al., 1986]

Na^+/K^+ ATPase
- Intestine [Montero and Ilundain, 1989]
- Liver [Häussinger et al., 1990c]
- Thick ascending limb [Hebert, 1986]

Cellular accumulation of amino acids [Bevan et al., 1990; Fincham et al., 1987; Fugelli and Rohrs, 1980; Hoffmann and Hendil, 1976; Hoffmann and Lambert, 1983; Kimelberg et al., 1990a; King and Goldstein, 1983; Law and Turner, 1987; Pasantes-Morales and Schousboe, 1988; Roy and Sauve, 1987; Sanchez Olea et al., 1991; Thurston et al., 1981; Vislie, 1983]

Cellular accumulation of polyoles [Garcia-Perez and Burg, 1990; Garty et al., 1991; Moriyama et al., 1990; Siebens and Spring, 1989; Yamauchi et al., 1991]

Cellular accumulation of methylamines [Garcia-Perez and Burg, 1990; Garty et al., 1991; Moriyama et al., 1990; Siebens and Spring, 1989; Yamauchi et al., 1991]

Net glycogenolysis [Baquet et al., 1990; Lang et al., 1989]

Net protein synthesis [Hallbrucker et al., 1991a; Häussinger et al., 1990a, b, 1991; Häussinger and Lang, 1991a, b]

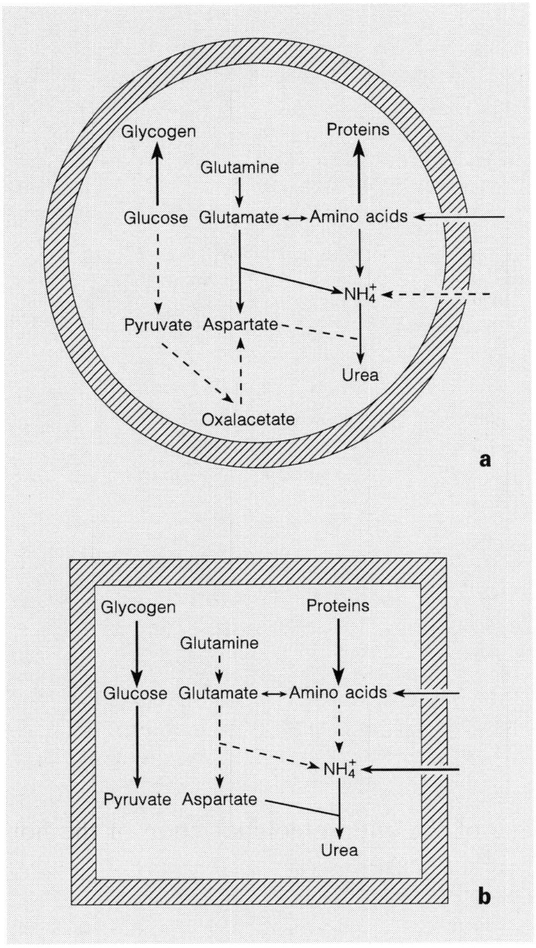

Fig. 3. Metabolic effects of cell swelling (**a**) and cell shrinkage (**b**); broken arrows indicate reduced flux, bold arrows enhanced flux [according to Häussinger and Lang, 1991c].

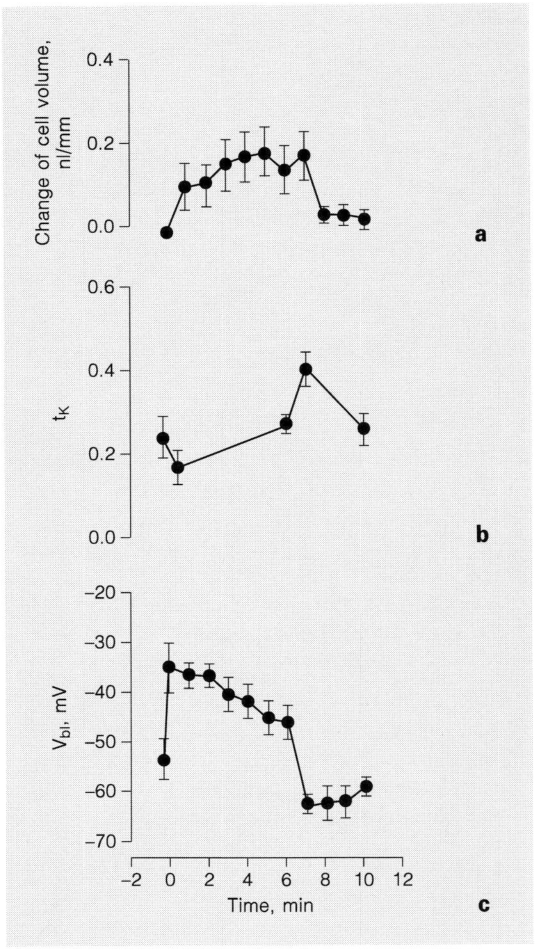

Fig. 4. Increase of cell volume (**a**) and alterations of K^+ conductance (**b**) and cell membrane potential (**c**) by transport of amino acids into proximal tubule cells [Beck and Potts, 1990; Lang et al., 1986].

Cell Volume and Cell Function

Epithelial Transport

In a variety of epithelia such as intestine, liver and kidney, transepithelial transport constitutes a major challenge for cell volume homeostasis. The sodium-coupled transport of organic substances such as amino acids and glucose, for example, leads to the cellular accumulation of osmotic activity, if the entry across the apical cell membrane surpasses the extrusion at the basolateral cell membrane. As a matter of fact, an increase of cell volume has been observed upon exposure of proximal tubule cells [Beck and Potts, 1990] and hepatocytes [Hallbrucker et al., 1991a] to amino acids. The cell swelling is expected to trigger cell volume regulatory mechanisms. Probably one of the consequences of cell swelling is the delayed activation of K^+ channels in the basolateral cell membrane of proximal tubules during stimulated sodium coupled transport [Lang and Rehwald, 1992]. This activation of K^+ channels leads to a hyperpolarization of the cell membranes and thus has further consequences for transepithelial transport (fig. 4). On the one hand, the hyperpolarization increases the electrical driving force and thus increases the sodium coupled transport. On the other hand, the hyperpolarization increases the electrical driving force for electrogenic bicarbonate exit across the basolateral cell membrane, thus leading to cellular acidification, to stimulation of the Na^+/H^+ antiporter and to enhanced transepithelial hydrogen ion secretion and bicarbonate reabsorption [Lang and Rehwald, 1992]. In the liver, cell volume does influence cellular uptake of amino acids [Häussinger and Lang, 1990)] as well as transepithelial taurocholate transport [Hallbrucker et al., 1992]. Thus, via their influence on cell volume, different transport systems could mutually influence each other.

Cell Volume in the Regulation of Hepatic Metabolism

As pointed out earlier (fig. 3), cell shrinkage stimulates net glycogenolysis and proteolysis and cell swelling stimulates net glycogen and protein synthesis. Thus, the consequences of cell swelling parallel effects of insulin and the consequences of cell shrinkage mimick effects of glucagon. Thus, we have tested for the possible participation of cell volume changes in the cellular mediation of the metabolic effects of these hormones [Hallbrucker et al., 1991b, c; Häussinger and Lang, 1991a–c]. As illustrated in figure 5, insulin does indeed lead to cell swelling and glucagon to cell shrinkage.

Insulin increases the cell volume by stimulation of the $Na^+,K^+,2Cl^-$ cotransporter and the Na^+/H^+ antiporter. Accordingly, the insulin-stimulated increment of cell volume is inhibited in part by furosemide or bumetanide and in part by amiloride. In the presence of both amiloride and furosemide the swelling effect of insulin is completely abolished.

Glucagon reduces the cell volume by activation of ion channels. Since glucagon depolarizes the cell membrane [unpubl. observation], the activation of anion channels appears to prevail. The action of glucagon on cell volume is mimicked and probably mediated by cAMP.

As apparent from figure 5, the effect of either hormone on cell volume fully accounts for its effect on proteolysis, i.e. the effect of the hormone is quantitatively mimicked by the respective osmotic alteration of cell volume and it is completely abolished following osmotic reversal of the cell volume change. Furosemide not only blunts the swelling effect of insulin but leads to a proportionate blunting of the antiproteolytic action of the hormone. Furthermore, induction of cell swelling by certain amino acids, such as glutamine and serine or by inhibition of K^+ channels with barium, leads to a similar antiproteolytic effect per change of cell volume as insulin.

Similarly, cell volume changes certainly do participate in the hormonal regulation of glycogen metabolism. However, at present we do not know to what extent cell volume changes account for the influence of insulin and glucagon on this and further metabolic functions. Nevertheless, it is appropriate to conclude that cell volume serves as a 'second messenger' mediating part of the cellular actions of insulin and glucagon [Häussinger and Lang, 1991c].

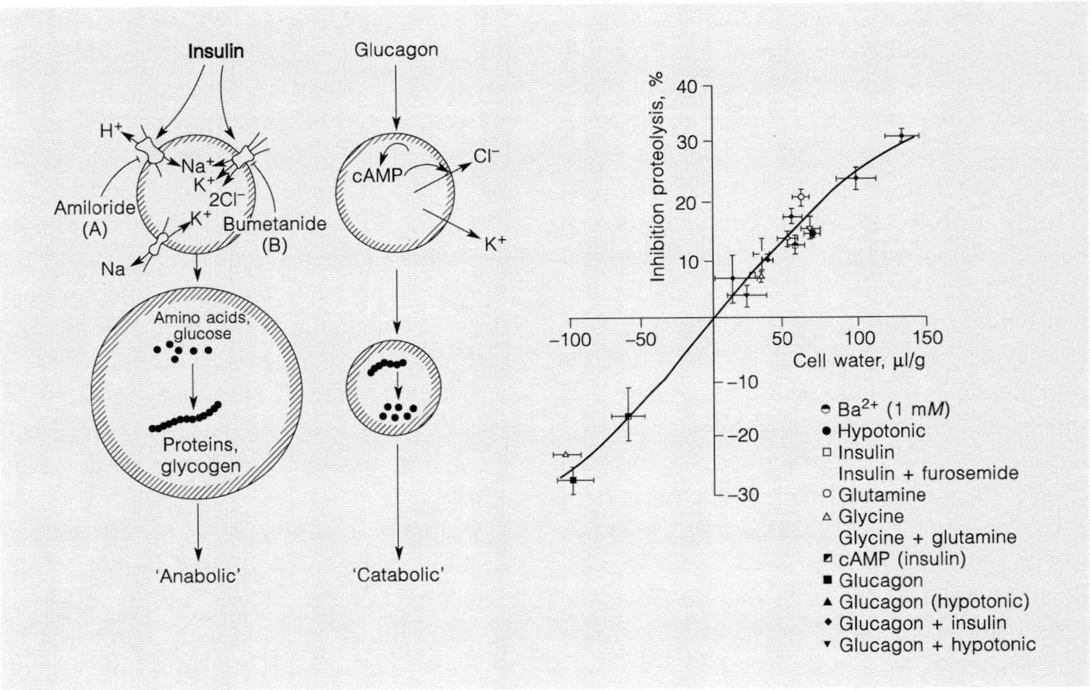

Fig. 5. Regulation of hepatic metabolism by insulin and glucagon via alterations of cell volume: insulin activates the $Na^+,K^+,2Cl^-$ cotransporter and the Na^+/H^+ antiporter. The cellular accumulation of electrolytes leads to cell swelling. Glucagon activates (via cAMP) a chloride and possibly a K^+ channel. The resulting cellular electrolyte loss leads to cell shrinkage. The alterations of cell volume are followed by the respective alterations of cell metabolism [according to Häussinger and Lang, 1991c].

Cell Volume and the Regulation of Cell Proliferation

For several years growth factors have been known to activate Na^+/H^+ antiport and $Na^+,K^+,2Cl^-$ cotransport [for a review, see Bianchini and Grinstein, 1992]. In the face of the above discussion, one obvious consequence of the activation of the two carriers is the increase of cell volume.

To test for an interaction of cell volume and cell proliferation we have studied cell proliferation and cell volume regulation in ras oncogene-expressing cells. The products of ras oncogenes are GTP binding proteins resistant to inactivation by GTPase [Barbacid, 1987]. Ras oncogenes are expressed in a variety of tumors and expression of ras oncogenes leads to transformation [Bishop, 1991].

As illustrated in figure 6, cell volume is markedly enhanced in cells expressing the ras oncogene. If exposed to anisotonic extracellular fluid, both ras oncogene expressing cells (+ras) and cells not expressing the ras oncogene (–ras) exhibit cell volume regulation. However, the set point of cell volume regulation is shifted to greater cell volumes in +ras.

Regulatory cell volume decrease is inhibited by quinidine and barium in both +ras and –ras and thus probably involves activation of

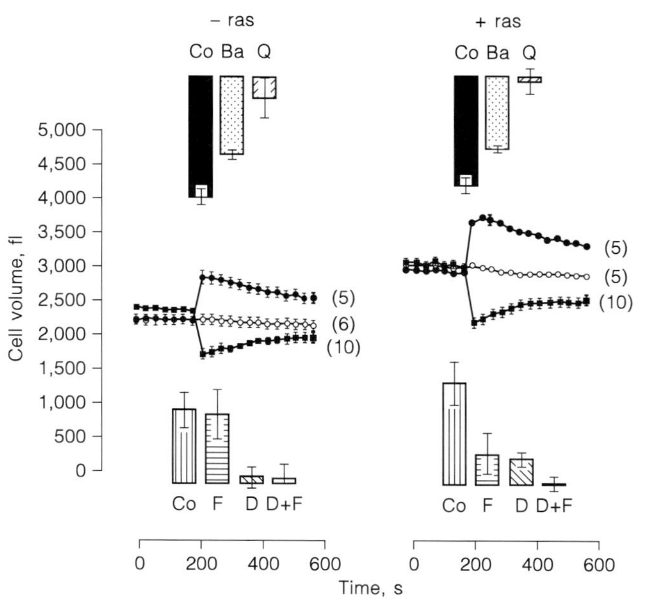

Fig. 6. Altered cell volume regulation in ras oncogene-expressing cells. In NIH fibroblasts the expression of ras oncogene leads to an increase of cell volume by some 40%. Exposure to anisotonic extracellular fluid leads to respective cell volume regulation in both cells expressing (+ras) and not expressing (–ras) the oncogene. However, the set point for cell volume regulation is shifted towards greater volumes in +ras [modified from Lang et al., 1992c].

ion channels. In –ras, regulatory cell volume increase is completely abolished by amiloride and not significantly affected by furosemide. In +ras, however, regulatory cell volume increase is only partially inhibited by amiloride and partially by furosemide or bumetanide. Only in the presence of both, amiloride and furosemide, regulatory cell volume increase is completely abolished. Accordingly, regulatory cell volume increase is probably accomplished by Na^+/H^+ antiport in –ras and by both Na^+/H^+ antiport and $Na^+,K^+,2Cl^-$ cotransport in +ras.

At present, we do not know, how cell volume interacts with cell proliferation. However, the growth factor-independent proliferation of +ras is abolished in the presence of furosemide, bumetanide or amiloride. Thus, activation of Na^+/H^+ antiport and of $Na^+,K^+,2Cl^-$ cotransport are apparently prerequisites for the proliferation of the ras oncogene-expressing cells.

Cell Volume in the Hepatic Regulation of Renal Function

As a last example, the possible role of cell volume for the hepatic regulation of renal function shall be illustrated. The potential influence of the liver on the kidneys has been a matter of debate for the past 3 decades [for a review, see Lang et al., 1992a]. One reason to believe that such an influence does exist is the prevalence of reversible renal failure in patients with hepatic disease, the so-called hepatorenal syndrome [Davidson and Dunn, 1987].

Since cell injury eventually leads to cell swelling, we hypothesized that it may be the liver cell swelling which triggers the hepatorenal syndrome. To test this hypothesis, we infused glutamine into the superior mesenteric vein in concentrations known to increase liver cell volume [Wettstein et al., 1990]. As a matter of fact glutamine leads indeed to a marked decrease of renal blood flow, renal glomerular

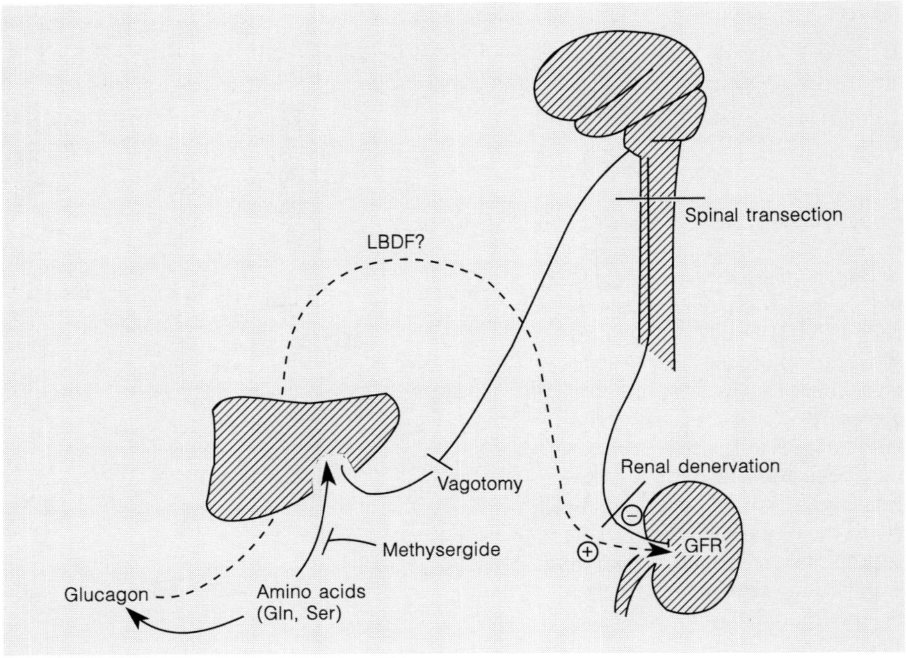

Fig. 7. Hepatic regulation of renal function. Portal venous infusion of amino acids glutamine (Gln) and serine (Ser) triggers a hepatorenal reflex decreasing renal glomerular filtration rate (GFR) and urinary flow rate (V). On the other hand, perivascular nerve stimulation at the portal vein as well as portal venous infusion of adenosine or glucagon leads probably via humoral factor(s) – 'liver-borne diuretic factor(s) (LBDF)' – to an increase of GFR and V. The reflex and the release of the LBDF may be sensitive to hepatic cellular volume [modified from Lang et al., 1992a].

filtration rate and urinary flow rate. The infusion of identical amounts of glutamine into the jugular vein did not elicit any of these effects [Lang et al., 1991a]. The effect of mesenteric glutamine was abolished by hepatic vagal or renal denervation or transection of the spinal cord at the thoracocervical junction [Lang et al., 1991a], it was inhibited by the serotonin antagonist methysergide and was mimicked by serotonin [Lang et al., 1991b]. Thus, we have concluded that mesenteric glutamine modifies renal function by triggering a serotoninergic hepatorenal reflex [Lang et al., 1991b]. At first glance, this observation contrasts the hyperfiltrative effect of amino acids. However, the effect of glutamine is reversed by glucagon, which is released by amino acids and decreases liver cell volume [Hallbrucker et al., 1991b; Lang et al., 1991a]. The effect of glucagon is not abolished by transection of the spinal cord and is thus not likely to be mediated via a hepatorenal reflex. Glucagon rather acts by stimulating the hepatic release of a humoral factor (fig. 7). The existence of a hepatic 'glomerulopressin' has been postulated earlier by Uranga et al. [1979a, b].

It should be pointed out that the evidence for the involvement of cell volume in the triggering of the hepatorenal reflex and the release of the liver-borne diuretic factor is circumstantial. Nevertheless, the experiments revealed powerful mechanisms of hepatorenal regulation and are at least suggestive for the involvement of liver cell volume.

Conclusions and Future Perspectives

The ability to regulate their volume belongs to the elementary requirements for the survival of cells. Thus, cells have developed a machinery of cell volume regulatory mechanisms comprising solute transport across the cell membrane and metabolism. Hormones such as insulin, glucagon and growth factors utilize the volume regulatory mechanisms to exert their effects on cellular function. Accordingly, the cell volume regulatory mechanisms are an integral part of the intracellular cascade transmitting hormonal signals. Furthermore, circumstantial evidence points to the involvement of cell volume in integrative functions such as the regulation of renal function by the liver.

The most intriguing goals for future research appear to be the identification of the mechanisms linking cell volume to the ion channels and carriers at the cell membrane as well as to metabolic activity of the cell. Furthermore, the search for the liver-borne diuretic factor(s) promises new insight into the interorgan regulation of salt and water balance.

References

Adorante, J.S.; Miller, S.S.: Potassium-dependent volume regulation in retinal pigment epithelium is mediated by Na,K,Cl cotransport. J. gen. Physiol. *96:* 1153–1176 (1990).

Adragna, N.C.; Tosteson, D.C.: Effect of volume changes on ouabain-insensitive net outward cation movements in human red cells. J. Membr. Biol. *78:* 43–52 (1984).

Bakker-Grunwald, T.: Hormone-induced diuretic-sensitive potassium transport in turkey erythrocytes is anion dependent. Biochim. biophys. Acta *641:* 427–431 (1981).

Bakker-Grunwald T.; Ogden, P.; Lamb, J.F.: Effects of ouabain and osmolarity on bumetanide-sensitive potassium transport in simian virus-transformed 3T3 cells. Biochim. biophys. Acta *687:* 333–336 (1982).

Ballanyi, K.; Grafe, P.: Cell volume regulation in the nervous system. Renal Physiol. Biochem. *11:* 142–157 (1988).

Baquet, A.; Hue, L.; Meijer, A.J.; Woerkom, G.M., van; Plomp, P.J.A.M.: Swelling of rat hepatocytes stimulates glycogen synthesis. J. biol. Chem. *265:* 955–959 (1990).

Barbacid, M.: ras genes. Annu. Rev. Biochem. *56:* 779–827 (1987).

Beck, F.-X.; Dörge, A.; Thurau, K.: Cellular osmoregulation in renal medulla. Renal Physiol. Biochem. *11:* 174–186 (1988).

Beck, F.-X.; Dörge, A.; Thurau, K.; Guder, W.: Cell osmoregulation in the countercurrent system of the renal medulla. Comp. Physiol. *4:* 132–158 (1990).

Beck, F.X.; Potts, D.J.: Cell swelling, co-transport activation and potassium conductance in isolated perfused rabbit kidney proximal tubules. J. Physiol. *425:* 369–378 (1990).

Beebe, D.C.; Parmelee, J.T.; Belcher, K.S.: Volume regulation in lens epithelial cells and differentiating lens fiber cells. J. cell. Physiol. *143:* 455–459 (1990).

Bevan, C.; Theiss, C.; Kinne, R.K.H.: The role of Ca^{2+} in sorbitol release from rat inner medullary collecting duct (IMCD) cells under hypoosmotic stress. Biochem. Biophys. Res. Commun. *170:* 563–568 (1990).

Bianchini, L.; Grinstein, S.: Regulation of volume-modulating ion transport systems by growth promoters. Adv. comp. Env. (1993, in press).

Bishop, J.M.: Molecular themes in oncogenesis. Cell *64:* 235–248 (1991).

Blumenfeld, J.D.; Hebert, S.C.; Heilig, C.W.; Balschi, J.A.; Stromski, M.E.; Gullans, S.R.: Organic osmolytes in inner medulla of Brattleboro rat: effects of ADH and dehydration. Am. J. Physiol. *256:* F916–F922 (1989).

Bonanno, J.A.: K^+–H^+ exchange, a fundamental cell acidifier in corneal epithelium. Am. J. Physiol. *260:* C618–C625 (1991).

Butt, A.G.; Clapp, W.L.; Frizzell, R.A.: Potassium conductance in tracheal epithelium activated by secretion and cell swelling. Am. J. Physiol. *258:* C630–C638 (1990).

Cala, P. M.: Volume regulation by Amphiuma red blood cells. The membrane potential and its implications regarding the nature of the ion-flux pathways. J. gen. Physiol. *76:* 683–708 (1980).
Cala, P. M.: Cell volume regulation by Amphiuma red blood cells. The role of Ca^{2+} as a modulator of alkali metal/H^+ exchange. J. gen. Physiol. *82:* 761–784 (1983).
Cala, P. M.: Volume regulation by Amphiuma red blood cells: characteristics of volume-sensitive K/H and Na/H exchange. Molec. Physiol. *8:* 199–214 (1985).
Cala, P. M.; Mandel, L. J.; Murphy, E.: Volume regulation by Amphiuma red blood cells: cytosolic free Ca and alkali metal-H exchange. Am. J. Physiol. *250:* C423–C429 (1986).
Chamberlin, M. E.; Strange, K.: Anti-osmotic cell volume regulation: a comparative view. Am. J. Physiol. *257:* C159–C173 (1989).
Chassande, O., Frelin, C.; Farahifar, D.; Jean, T.; Lazduski, M.: The Na^+,K^+,2 Cl^- cotransport in C6 glioma cells. Properties and role in volume regulation. Eur. J. Biochem. *171:* 425–433 (1988).
Cheung, R. K.; Grinstein, S.; Dosch, H.-M.; Gelfand, E.W.: Volume regulation by human lymphocytes: characterization of the ionic basis for regulatory volume decrease. J. cell. Physiol. *112:* 189–196 (1982).
Christensen, O.: Mediation of cell volume regulation by Ca^{2+} influx through stretch-activated channels. Nature *330:* 66–68 (1987).
Christensen, O.; Simon, M.; Randlev, T.: Anion channels in a leaky epithelium. A patch clamp study of choroid plexus. Pflügers Arch. *415:* 37–46 (1989).
Costa, P. M.; Fernandes, P. L.; Ferreira, H. G.; Ferreira, K.T.; Giraldez, F.: Effect of cell volume changes on membrane ionic permeabilities and sodium transport in frog skin *(Rana ridibunda)*. J. Physiol. *393:* 1–17 (1987).
Davidson, E.W.; Dunn, M. J.: Pathogenesis of the hepatorenal syndrome. Annu. Rev. Med. *38:* 361–372 (1987).
Davis, C.W.; Finn, A. L.: Cell volume regulation in frog urinary bladder. Fed. Proc. *44:* 2520–2525 (1985).
Davis, C.W.; Finn, A. L.: Interactions of sodium transport, cell volume, and calcium in frog urinary bladder. J. gen. Physiol. *89:* 687–702 (1987).
Deutsch, C.; Lee, S. C.: Cell volume regulation in lymphocytes. Renal Physiol. Biochem. *11:* 260–276 (1988).
Donaldson, P. J.; Chen, L. K.; Lewis, S. A.: Effects of serosal anion composition on the permeability properties of rabbit urinary bladder. Am. J. Physiol. *256:* F1125–F1134 (1989).
Drewnowska, K.; Baumgarten, C. M.: Regulation of cellular volume in rabbit ventricular myocytes: bumetanide, chlorothiazide, and ouabain. Am. J. Physiol. *260:* C122–C131 (1991).
Duhm, J.; Göbel, B. O.: Na^+–K^+ transport and volume of rat erythrocytes under dietary K^+ deficiency. Am. J. Physiol. *246:* 246: C20–C29 (1984).
Dunham, P. B.; Ellory, J. C.: Passive potassium transport in low potassium sheep red cells: dependence upon cell volume and chloride. J. Physiol. *318:* 511–530 (1981).
Ellory, J. C.; Hall, A. C.; Stewart, G.W.: Volume-sensitive cation fluxes in mammalian red cells. Molec. Physiol. *8:* 235–246 (1985).
Ericson, A.-C.; Spring, K. R.: Volume regulation by Necturus gallbladder: apical Na^+–H^+ and Cl^-–HCO_3^- exchange. Am. J. Physiol. *243:* C146–C150 (1982).
Eveloff, J. L.; Calamia, J.: Effect of osmolarity on cation fluxes in medullary thick ascending limb cells. Am. J. Physiol. *250:* F176–F180 (1986).
Farahbakhsh, N. A.; Fain, G. L.: Volume regulation of non-pigmented cells from ciliary epithelium. Invest. Ophthalmol. vis. Sci. *28:* 934–944 (1987).
Fincham, D. A.; Wolowyk, M.W.; Young, J. D.: Volume-sensitive taurine transport in fish erythrocytes. J. Membr. Biol. *96:* 45–56 (1987).
Finn, A. L.; Reuss, L.: Effects of changes in the ionic composition of the serosal solution on the electrical properties of the toad urinary bladder epithelium. J. Physiol. *250:* 541–558 (1975).
Fisher, R. S.; Persson, B. E.; Spring, K. R.: Epithelial cell-volume regulation: bicarbonate dependence. Science *214:* 1357–1359 (1981).
Frelin, C.; Chassande, O.; Lazdunski, M.: Biochemical characterization of the $Na^+/K^+/2Cl^-$ co-transport in chick cardiac cells. Biochem. biophys. Res. Commun. *134:* 326–331 (1986).
Fugelli, K.; Rohrs, H.: The effect of Na^+ and osmolality the on influx and steady state distribution of taurine and gamma-aminobutyric acid in flounder *(Platichthys flesus)* erythrocytes. Compar. Biochem. Physiol. *67A:* 545–551 (1980).
Garcia-Perez, A.; Burg, M. B.: Importance of organic osmolytes for osmoregulation by renal medullary cells. Hypertension *16:* 595–602 (1990).
Garcia-Perez, A.; Burg, M. B.: Role of organic osmolytes in adaptation of renal cells to high osmolality. J. Membr. Biol. *119:* 1–13 (1991).
Garty, H.; Furlong, T. J.; Ellis, D. E.; Spring, K. R.: Sorbitol permease: an apical membrane transporter in cultured renal papillary epithelial cells. Am. J. Physiol. *260:* F650–F656 (1991).
Geck, P.; Pietrzyk, C.; Burckhardt, B.-C.; Pfeiffer, B.; Heinz, E.: Electrically silent cotransport of Na^+, K^+ and Cl^- in Ehrlich cells. Biochim. biophys. Acta *600:* 432–447 (1980).
Geck, P.; Heinz, E.: The Na-K-2Cl cotranport system. J. Membr. Biol. *91:* 97–105 (1986).
Geck, P.: Volume regulation in Ehrlich cells. Comp. Physiol. *4:* 26–58 (1990).
Germann, W. J.; Ernst, S. A.; Dawson, D. C.: Resting and osmotically induced basolateral K conductances in turtle colon. J. gen. Physiol. *88:* 253–274 (1986).
Gilles, R.: Comparative aspects of cell osmoregulation and volume control. Renal Physiol. Biochem. *11:* 277–288 (1988).
Graf, J.; Haddad, P.; Häussinger, D.; Lang, F.: Cell volume regulation in liver. Renal Physiol. Biochem. *11:* 202–220 (1988).

Graf, J.; Guggino, W.B.; Turnheim, K.: Volume regulation in transporting epithelia. Adv. comp. Env. Physiol. (1992, in press).

Green, J.; Yamaguchi, D.T.; Kleeman, C.R.; Muallem, S.: Selective modification of the kinetic properties of Na^+/H^+ exchanger by cell shrinkage and swelling. J. biol. Chem. *263:* 5012–5015 (1988).

Grinstein, S.; Clarke, C.A.; Rothstein, A.: Increased anion permeability during volume regulation in human lymphocytes. Phil. Trans. R. Soc. Lond. *B299:* 509–518 (1982a).

Grinstein, S.; Dupre, A.; Rothstein, A.: Volume regulation by human lymphocytes. Role of calcium. J. gen. Physiol. *79:* 849–868 (1982b).

Grinstein, S.; Clarke, C.A.; Dupre, A.; Rothstein, A.: Volume-induced increase of anion permeability in human lymphocytes. J. gen. Physiol. *80:* 801–823 (1982c).

Grinstein, S.; Clarke, C.A.; Rothstein, A.; Gelfand, E.W.: Volume-induced anion conductance in human B lymphocytes is cation independent. Am. J. Physiol. *245:* C160–C163 (1983a).

Grinstein, S.; Clarke, C.A.; Rothstein, A.: Activation of Na^+/H^+ exchange in lymphocytes by osmotically induced volume changes and by cytoplasmic acidification. J. gen. Physiol. *82:* 619–638 (1983b).

Grinstein, S.; Rothstein, A.; Sarkadi, B.; Gelfand, E.W.: Responses of lymphocytes to anisotonic media: volume-regulating behavior. Am. J. Physiol. *246:* C204–C215 (1984).

Grinstein, S.; Goetz, J.D.; Cohen, S.; Furuya, W.; Rothstein, A.; Gelfand, E.W.: Mechanism of regulatory volume increase in osmotically shrunken lymphocytes. Molec. Physiol. *8:* 185–198 (1985a).

Grinstein, S.; Rothstein, A.; Cohen, S.: Mechanism of osmotic activation of Na^+/H^+ exchange in rat thymic lymphocytes. J. gen. Physiol. *85:* 765–787 (1985b).

Halestrap, A.P.: The regulation of organelle function through changes in their volume. Adv. comp. Env. Physiol. (1992, in press).

Hallbrucker, C.; Vom Dahl, S.; Lang, F.; Häussinger, D.: Control of hepatic proteolysis by amino acids: the role of cell volume. Eur. J. Biochem. *197:* 717–724 (1991a).

Hallbrucker, C.; Vom Dahl, S.; Lang, F.; Gerok, W.; Häussinger, D.: Inhibition of hepatic proteolysis by insulin: role of hormone induced alterations of cellular K^+ balance. Eur. J. Biochem. *199:* 467–474 (1991b).

Hallbrucker, C.; Vom Dahl, S.; Lang, F.; Gerok, W.; Häussinger, D.: Modification of liver cell volume by insulin and glucagon. Pflügers Arch. *418:* 519–521 (1991c).

Hallbrucker, C.; Lang, F.; Häussinger, D.: Cell volume is a major factor regulating biliary taurocholate excretion. Hepatology (1992, in press).

Häussinger, D.; Lang, F.: Exposure of perfused liver to hypotonic conditions modifies cellular nitrogen metabolism. J. cell. Biochem. *43:* 355–361 (1990).

Häussinger, D.; Hallbrucker, C.; Vom Dahl, S.; Lang, F.; Gerok, W.: Cell swelling inhibits proteolysis in perfused rat liver. Biochem. J. *272:* 239–242 (1990a).

Häussinger, D.; Lang, F.; Bauers, K.; Gerok, W.: Control of hepatic nitrogen metabolism and glutathione release by cell volume regulatory mechanisms. Eur. J. Biochem. *193:* 891–898 (1990b).

Häussinger, D.; Stehle, T.; Lang, F.: Volume regulation in liver: further characterization by inhibitors and ionic substitutions. Hepatology. *11:* 243–254 (1990c).

Häussinger, D.; Hallbrucker, C.; Vom Dahl, S.; Decker, S.; Schweizer, U.; Lang, F.; Gerok, W.: Cell volume is a major determinant of proteolysis control in liver. FEBS Lett. *283:* 70–72 (1991).

Häussinger, D.; Lang, F.: The mutual interaction between cell volume and cell function: a new principle of metabolic regulation. Biochem. Cell Biol. *69:* 1–4 (1991a).

Häussinger, D.; Lang, F.: Cell volume in the regulation of hepatic function: a new mechanism for metabolic control. Biochim. biophys. Acta (1991b, in press).

Häussinger, D.; Lang, F.: Cell volume – a 'second messenger' in the regulation of metabolism by amino acids and hormones. Cell. Physiol. Biochem. *1:* 121–130 (1991c).

Häussinger, D.; Gerok, W.; Lang, F.: Cell volume and hepatic metabolism. Adv. comp. Env. Physiol. (1993, in press).

Hazama, A.; Okada, Y.: Ca^{2+} sensitivity of volume regulatory K^+ and Cl^- channels in cultured human epithelial cells. J. Physiol. *402:* 687–702 (1988).

Hebert, S.C.: Hypertonic cell volume regulation in mouse thick limbs. II. Na^+/H^+ and Cl^-/HCO_3^- exchange in basolateral membranes. Am. J. Physiol. *250:* C920–C931 (1986).

Hoffmann, E.K.; Hendil, K.B.: The role of amino acids and taurine in isomotic intracellular regulation in Ehrlich ascites mouse tumour cells. J. comp. Physiol. *108:* 279–286 (1976).

Hoffmann, E.K.; Lambert, I.H.: Amino acid transport and cell volume regulation in Ehrlich ascites tumour cells. J. Physiol. *338:* 613–625 (1983).

Hoffmann, E.K.; Sjoholm, C.; Simonsen, L.O.: Na^+,Cl^- cotransport in Ehrlich ascites tumor cells activated during volume regulation (regulatory volume increase). J. Membr. Biol. *76:* 269–280 (1983).

Hoffmann, E.K.; Simonsen, L.O.; Lambert, I.H.: Volume-induced increase of K^+ and Cl^- permeabilities in Ehrlich ascites tumor cells. Role of internal Ca^{2+}. J. Membr. Biol. *78:* 211–222 (1984).

Hoffmann, E.K.: Role of separate K^+ and Cl^- channels and of Na^+/Cl^- cotransport in volume regulation in Ehrlich cells. Fed. Proc. *44:* 2513–2519 (1985a).

Hoffmann, E.K.: Regulatory volume decrease in Ehrlich ascites tumor cells: role of inorganic ions and amino compounds. Molec. Physiol. *8:* 167–184 (1985b).

Hoffmann, E.K.; Lambert, I.H.; Simonsen, L.O.: Separate, Ca^{2+}-activated K^+ and Cl^- transport pathways in Ehrlich ascites tumor cells. J. Membr. Biol. *91:* 227–244 (1986).

Hoffmann, E.K.: Volume regulation in cultured cells. Curr. Top. Membr. Transp. *30:* 125–180 (1987).

Hoffmann, E.K.; Lambert, I.H.; Simonsen, L.O.: Mechanisms in volume regulation in Ehrlich ascites tumor cells. Renal Physiol. Biochem. *11:* 221–247 (1988).
Hoffmann, E.K.; Simonsen, L.O.: Membrane mechanisms in volume and pH regulation in vertebrate cells. Physiol. Rev. *69:* 315–382 (1989).
Hoffmann, E.K.; Simonsen, L.O.; Lambert, I.H.: Cell volume regulation: intracellular transmission. Adv. comp. Env. Physiol. (1993, in press).
Hudson, R.L.; Schultz, S.G.: Sodium-coupled glycine uptake by Ehrlich ascites tumor cells results in an increase in cell volume and plasma membrane channel activities. Proc. natn. Acad. Sci. USA *85:* 279–283 (1988).
Jennings, M.L.; Douglas, S.M.; McAndrew, P.E.: Amiloride-sensitive sodium-hydrogen exchange in osmotically shrunken rabbit red blood cells. Am. J. Physiol. *251:* C32–C40 (1986).
Kimelberg, H.K.; Frangakis, M.V.: Volume regulation in primary astrocyte cultures. Adv. Biosci. *61:* 177–186 (1986).
Kimelberg, H.K.; Goderie, S.K.; Higman, S.; Pang, S.; Waniewski, R.A.: Swelling-induced release of glutamate, aspartate, and taurine from astrocyte cultures. J. Neurosci. *10:* 1583–1591 (1990a).
Kimelberg, H.K.; Anderson, E.; Kettenmann, H.: Swelling induced changes in electrophysiological properties of cultured astrocytes and oligodendrocytes. II. Whole cell currents. Brain Res. *529:* 262–268 (1990b).
Kimelberg, H.K.; Kettenmann, H.: Swelling-induced changes in electrophysiological properties of cultured astrocytes and oligodendrocytes. I. Effects on membrane potentials, input impedance and cell-cell coupling. Brain Res. *529:* 255–261 (1990).
Kimelberg, H.K.; O'Connor, E.R.; Kettenmann, H.: Effects of swelling on glial cell function. Adv. comp. Env. Physiol. (1993, in press).
King, P.A.; Goldstein, L.: Organic osmolytes and cell volume regulation in fish. Mol. Physiol. *4:* 53–66 (1983).
Kirk, K.L.; DiBona, D.R.; Schafer, J.A.: Regulatory volume decrease in perfused proximal nephron: evidence for a dumping of cell K^+. Am. J. Physiol. *252:* F933–F942 (1987a).
Kirk, K.L.; Schafer, J.A.; DiBona, D.R.: Cell volume regulation in rabbit proximal straight tubule perfused in vitro. Am. J. Physiol. *252:* F922–F932 (1987b).
Kleinzeller, A.; Ziyadeh, F.N.: Volume regulation in epithelia. Comp. Physiol. *4:* 59–86 (1990).
Kramhoft, B., Lambert, I.H.; Hoffmann, E.K.; Jorgensen F.: Activation of Cl-dependent K transport in Ehrlich ascites tumor cells. Am. J. Physiol. *251:* C369–C379 (1986).
Kregenow, F.M.: Osmoregulatory salt transporting mechanisms: control of cell volume in anisotonic media. Annu. Rev. Physiol. *43:* 493–505 (1981).
Kregenow, F.M.; Caryk, T.; Siebens, A.W.: Further studies of the volume-regulatory response of Amphiuma red cells in hypertonic media. Evidence for amiloride-sensitive Na/H exchange. J. gen. Physiol. *86:* 565–584 (1985).
Kristensen, L.O.; Folke, M.: Volume-regulatory K^+ efflux during concentrative uptake of alanine in isolated rat hepatocytes. Biochem. J. *221:* 265–268 (1984).
Kristensen, L.O.: Associations between transports of alanine and cations across cell membrane in rat hepatocytes. Am. J. Physiol. *251:* G575–G584 (1986).
Kurtz, A.; Scholz, H.: Cell volume and stimulus-secretion coupling. Adv. comp. Env. Physiol. (1993, in press).
Lambert, I.H.: Effect of arachidonic acid, fatty acids, prostaglandins, and leukotrienes on volume regulation in Ehrlich ascites tumor cells. J. Membr. Biol. *98:* 207–221 (1987).
Lang, F.; Messner, G.; Rehwald, W.: Electrophysiology of sodium-coupled transport in proximal renal tubules. Am. J. Physiol. *250:* F953–F962 (1986).
Lang, F.; Paulmichl, M.; Völkl, H.; Gstrein, E.; Friedrich, F.: Electrophysiology of cell volume regulation; in Kovacevic, Guder, Molecular physiology: biochemical aspects of kidney function, pp.133–139 (de Gruyter, Berlin 1987).
Lang, F.; Stehle, T.; Häussinger, D.: Water, K^+, H^+, lactate and glucose fluxes during cell volume regulation in perfused rat liver. Pflügers Arch. *413:* 209–216 (1989).
Lang, F.; Friedrich, F.; Paulmichl, M.; Schobersberger, W.; Jungwirth, A.; Ritter, M.; Steidl, M.; Weiss, H.; Wöll, E.; Tschernko, E.; Paulmichl, R.; Hallbrucker, C.: Ion channels in Madin-Darby canine kidney cells. Renal Physiol. Biochem. *13:* 82–93 (1990).
Lang, F.; Tschernko, E.; Schulze, E.; Öttl, I.; Ritter, M.; Völkl, H.; Hallbrucker, C.; Häussinger, D.: Hepatorenal reflex regulating kidney function. Hepatology *14:* 590–594 (1991a).
Lang, F.; Öttl, I.; Freudenschuss, K.; Honeder, M.; Tschernko, E.; Häussinger, D.: Serotoninergic hepatorenal reflex regulating renal glomerular filtration rate. Pflügers Arch. *419:* 111–113 (1991b).
Lang, F.; Rehwald, W.: Potassium channels in renal epithelial transport regulation. Physiol. Rev. *20:* 1–39 (1992).
Lang, F.; Häussinger, D.; Tschernko, E.; Capasso, G.; De Santo, N.G.: Proteins, the liver and the kidney – hepatic regulation of renal function. Nephron *61:* 1–4 (1992a).
Lang, F.; Ritter, M.; Völkl, H.; Häussinger, D.: Cell volume regulatory mechanisms – an overview. Adv. comp. Env. Physiol. (1993b, in press).
Lang, F.; Ritter, M.; Wöll, E.; Weiss, H.; Häussinger, D.; Maly, K.; Grunicke, H.: Altered cell volume regulation in ras oncogene expressing NIH fibroblasts. Pflügers Arch. *420:* 424–427 (1992c).
Lapointe, J.Y.; Garneau, L.; Bell, P.D.; Cardinal, J.: Membrane crosstalk in the proximal tubule during alterations in transepithelial sodium transport. Am. J. Physiol. *258:* F339–F345 (1990).

Larson, M.; Spring, K.R.: Volume regulation by Necturus gallbladder: basolateral KCl exit. J. Membr. Biol. 81: 219–232 (1984).
Lau, K.R., Hudson, R.L.; Schultz, S.G.: Cell swelling increases a barium-inhibitable potassium conductance in the basolateral membrane of Necturus small intestine. Proc. natn. Acad. Sci. USA *81:* 3591–3594 (1984).
Lauf, P.K.: Evidence for chloride dependent potassium and water transport induced by hyposmotic stress in erythrocytes of the marine teleost, *Opsanus tau*. J. comp. Physiol. *146:* 9–16 (1982).
Lauf, P.K.: On the relationship between volume- and thiol-stimulated K^+ Cl^- fluxes in red cell membranes. Molec. Physiol. *8:* 215–234 (1985).
Lauf, P.K.: K:Cl cotransport: emerging molecular aspects of a ouabain-resistant, volume-responsive transport system in red blood cells. Renal Physiol. *11:* 248–259 (1988).
Law, R.O.; Turner, D.P.J.: Are ninhydrin-positive substances volume-regulatory osmolytes in rat renal papillary cells? J. Physiol. *386:* 24–51 (1987).
Leibowich, S.; DeLong, J.; Civan, M.M.: Apical Na^+ permeability of frog skin during serosal Cl^- replacement. J. Membr. Biol. *102:* 121–130 (1988).
Lewis, S.A.; Butt, A.G.; Bowler, M.J.; Leader, J.P.; Macknight, A.D.C.: Effects of anions on cellular volume and transepithelial Na^+ transport across toad urinary bladder. J. Membr. Biol. *83:* 119–137 (1985).
Livne, A.; Grinstein, S.; Rothstein, A.: Volume-regulating behavior of human platelets. J. cell. Physiol. *131:* 354–363 (1987).
Lohr, J.W.; Sullivan, L.P.; Cragoe, E.J.; Grantham, J.J.: Volume regulation determinants in isolated proximal tubules in hypertonic medium. Am. J. Physiol. *256:* F622–F631 (1989).
Macknight, A.D.C.; Leaf, A.: Regulation of cellular volume. Physiol. Rev. *57:* 510–573 (1977).
Macknight, A.D.C.: Volume maintenance in isosmotic conditions. Curr. Top. Membr. Transp. *30:* 3–43 (1987).
Macknight, A.D.C.: Principles of cell volume regulation. Renal Physiol. Biochem. *11:* 114–141 (1988).
MacLeod, R.J.; Hamilton, J.R.: Regulatory volume increase in isolated mammlian jejunal villus is due to bumetanide-sensitive $NaKCl_2$ cotransport. Am. J. Physiol. *258:* G665–G674 (1990).
McCann, J.D.; Li, M.; Welsh, M.J.: Identification and regulation of whole-cell chloride currents in airway epithelium. J. gen. Physiol. *94:* 1015–1036 (1989).
Mercer, R.W.; Hoffman, J.F.: Bumetanide-sensitive Na/K cotransport in ferret red blood cells (abstract). Biophys. J. *47:* 157a (1985).
Montero, M.C.; Ilundáin, A.: Effects of anisosmotic buffers on K^+ transport in isolated chicken enterocytes. Biochim. biophys. Acta *979:* 269–271 (1989).
Montrose, M.H.; Knoblauch, C.; Murer, H.: Separate control of regulatory volume increase and Na^+–H^+ exchange by cultured renal cells. Am. J. Physiol. *255:* C76–C85 (1988).
Moriyama, T.; Garcia-Perez, A.; Burg, M.B.: Factors affecting the ratio of different organic osmolytes in renal medullary cells. Am. J. Physiol. *259:* F847–F858 (1990).
Muallem, S.; Loessberg, P.A.: Intracellular pH-regulatory mechanisms in pancreatic acinar cells. II. Regulation of H^+ and HCO_3^- transporters by Ca^{2+}-mobilizing agonists. J. biol. Chem. *265:* 12813–12819 (1990).
Musch, M.W.; Field, M.: K-independent Na-Cl cotransport in bovine tracheal epithelial cells. Am. J. Physiol. *256:* C658–C665 (1989).
O'Neill, W.C.: Volume-sensitive Cl-dependent K transport in human erythrocytes. Am. J. Physiol. *253:* C883–C888 (1987).
O'Neill, W.C.; Mikkelsen, R.B.: Furosemide-sensitive Na^+ and K^+ transport and human erythrocyte volume. Biochim. biophys. Acta *896:* 196–202 (1987).
O'Neill, W.C.; Klein, J.D.: Regulation of vascular endothelial cell volume by Na-K-2Cl cotransport. Am. J. Physiol. (1992, in press).
O'Neill, W.C.: Cell volume regulation and vascular endothelial function. Adv. comp. Env. Physiol. (1993, in press).
Parker, J.C.; Gitelman, H.J.; Glosson, P.S.; Leonard, D.L.: Role of calcium in volume regulation by dog red blood cells. J. gen. Physiol. *65:* 84–95 (1974).
Parker, J.C.: Sodium and calcium movements in dog red blood cells. J. gen. Physiol. *71:* 1–17 (1978).
Parker, J.C.: Active and passive Ca movements in dog red blood cells and resealed ghosts. Am. J. Physiol. *237:* C10–C16 (1979).
Parker, J.C.: Hemolytic action of potassium salts on dog red blood cells. Am. J. Physiol. *244:* C313–C317 (1983a).
Parker, J.C.: Volume-responsive sodium movements in dog red blood cells. Am. J. Physiol. *244:* C324–C330 (1983b).
Parker, J.C.; Castranova, V.: Volume-responsive sodium and proton movements in dog red blood cells. J. gen. Physiol. *84:* 379–401 (1984).
Pasantes-Morales, H.; Schousboe, A.: Volume regulation in astrocytes: a role for taurine as osmoeffector. J. Neurosci. Res. *20:* 505–509 (1988).
Paulmichl, M.; Friedrich, F.; Maly, K.; Lang, F.: The effect of hypoosmolarity on the electrical properties of Madin-Darby canine kidney cells. Pflügers Arch. *413:* 456–462 (1989).
Reuss, L.: Independence of apical membrane Na^+ and Cl^- entry in Necturus gallbladder epithelium. J. gen. Physiol. *84:* 423–445 (1984).
Reuss, L.: Cell volume regulation in non-renal epithelia. Renal Physiol. Biochem. *11:* 187–201 (1988).
Ritter, M.; Paulmichl, M.; Lang, F.: Further characterization of volume regulatory decrease in cultured renal epitheloid (MDCK) cells. Pflügers Arch. *418:* 35–39 (1991a).
Ritter, M.; Steidl, M.; Lang, F.: Inhibition of ion conductances by osmotic shrinkage of Madin Darby canine kidney cells. Am. J. Physiol. *261:* C602–C607 (1991b).

Roy, G., Sauvé, R.: Effect of anisotonic media on volume, ion and amino-acid content and membrane potential of kidney cells (MDCK) in culture. J. Membr. Biol. *100:* 83–96 (1987).
Rugolo, M.; Mastocola, T.; Flamigni, A.; Lenaz, G.: Chloride transport in human fibroblasts is activated by hypotonic shock. Biochem. biophys. Res. Commun. *160:* 1330–1338 (1989).
Sackin, H.: Stretch-activated potassium channels in renal proximal tubule. Am. J. Physiol. *253:* F1253–F1262 (1987).
Sackin, H.: A stretch-activated K^+ channel sensitive to cell volume. Proc. natn. Acad. Sci. USA *86:* 1731–1735 (1989).
Sànchez Olea, R.; Pasantes-Morales, H.; Lázaro, A.; Cereijido, M.: Osmolarity-sensitive release of free amino acids from cultured kidney cells (MDCK). J. Membr. Biol. *121:* 1–9 (1991).
Sardet, C.; Counillon, L.; Franchi, A.; Pouyssegur, J.: Growth factors induce phosphorylation of the Na^+/H^+ antiporter, a glycoprotein of 110 kD. Science *247:* 723–726 (1990).
Sardet, C.; Wakayabashi, S.; Fafournoux, P.; Counillon, L.; Pages, G.; Pouyssegur, J.: Molecular properties of the Na^+/H^+ exchange; in De Santo, Capasso, Acid-base balance: molecular, cellular and clinical aspects, pp 13–20 (Editoriale Bios, Cosenza 1991).
Sarkadi, B.; Mack, E.; Rothstein, A.: Ionic events during the volume response of human peripheral blood lymphocytes to hypotonic media. I. Distinctions between volume-activated Cl^- and K^+ conductance pathways. J. gen. Physiol. *83:* 497–512 (1984a).
Sarkadi, B.; Mack, E.; Rothstein, A.: Ionic events during the volume response of human peripheral blood lymphocytes to hypotonic media. II. Volume- and time-dependent activation and inactivation of ion transport pathways. J. gen. Physiol. *83:* 513–527 (1984b).
Sarkadi, B.; Cheung, R.; Mack, E.; Grinstein, S.; Gelfand, E.W.; Rothstein, A.: Cation and anion transport pathways in volume regulatory response of human lymphocytes to hyposmotic media. Am. J. Physiol. *248:* C480–C487 (1985).
Schild, L.; Aronson, P.S.; Giebisch, G.: Basolateral transport pathways for K^+ and Cl^- in rabbit proximal tubule: effects on cell volume. Am. J. Physiol. *260:* F101–F109 (1991).
Schmidt, W.F. III; McManus, T.J.: Ouabain-insensitive salt and water movements in duck red cells. I. Kinetics of cation transport under hypotonic conditions. J. gen. Physiol. *70:* 59–79 /1977a).
Schmidt, W.F. III; McManus, T.J.: Ouabain-insensitive salt and water movements in duck red cells. II. Norepinephrine stimulation of sodium plus potassium cotransport. J. gen. Physiol. *70:* 81–97 (1977b).
Schmidt, W.F. III; McManus, T.J.: Ouabain-insensitive salt and water movements in duck red cells. III. The role of chloride in the volume response. J. gen. Physiol. *70:* 99–121 (1977c).
Schultz, S.G.; Hudson, R.L.; Lapointe, J.Y.: Electrophysiological studies of sodium cotransport in epithelia: towards a cellular model; in Semenza, Kinne, Membrane transport driven by ion gradients. Ann. N.Y. Acad. Sci. *456:* 127–135 (1985).
Schultz, S.G.: Volume preservation: then and now. News Physiol. Sci. *4:* 169–172 (1989).
Sernka, T.J.: Direct hyposmotic stimulation of gastric acid secretion. Membr. Biochem. *9:* 1–7 (1990).
Siebens, A.W.; Kregenow, F.M.: Volume-regulatory responses of Amphiuma red cells in anisotonic media. The effect of amiloride. J. gen. Physiol. *86:* 527–564 (1985).
Siebens, A.W.; Spring, K.R.: A novel sorbitol transport mechanism in cultured renal papillary epithelial cells. Am. J. Physiol. *257:* F937–F946 (1989).
Simmons, N.L.: Epithelial cell volume regulation in hypotonic fluids: studies using a model tissue culture renal epithelial cell system. Q. Jl. exp. Physiol. *69:* 83–95 (1984).
Soltoff, S.P.; McMillian, M.K.; Cantley, L.C.; Cragoe, E.J., Jr.; Talamo, B.R.: Effects of muscarinic, alpha-adrenergic, and substance P agonists and ionomycin on ion transport mechanisms in the rat parotid acinar cell. The dependence of ion transport on intracellular calcium. J. gen. Physiol. *93:* 285–319 (1989).
Spring, K.R.: Determinants of epithelial cell volume. Fed. Proc. *44:* 2526–2529 (1985).
Stoddard, J.S.; Reuss, L.: Electrophysiological effects of mucosal Cl^- removal in Necturus gallbladder epithelium. Am. J. Physiol. *257:* C568–C578 (1989).
Sun, A.; Hebert, S.C.: Rapid hypertonic cell volume regulation in the perfused inner medullary collecting duct. Kidney int. *36:* 831–842 (1989).
Tas, P.W.L.: Massa, P.T.; Kress, H.G.; Koschel, K.: Characterization of an $Na^+/K^+/Cl^-$ co-transport in primary cultures of rat astrocytes. Biochim. biophys. Acta *903:* 411–416 (1987).
Tauc, M.; Le Maout, S.; Poujeol, P.: Fluorescent videomicroscopy study of regulatory volume decrease in primary culture of rabbit proximal convoluted tubule. Biochim. biophys. Acta *1052:* 278–284 (1990).
Thurston, J.H.; Hauhart, R.E.; Naccarato, E.F.: Taurine: possible role in osmotic regulation of mammalian heart. Science *214:* 1373–1374 (1981).
Tivey, D.R.; Simmons, N.L.; Aiton, J.F.: Role of passive potassium fluxes in cell volume regulation in cultured HeLa cells. J. Membr. Biol. *85:* 93–105 (1985).
Uranga, J.; del Castillo, E.; Gimeno, M.: Action of glomerulopressin on smooth muscle contraction, probably mediated by the release of prostaglandins. Archs int. Phharmacodyn. *238:* 19–27 (1979a).
Uranga, J.; Fuenzalida, R.; Rapoport, A.L.; del Castillo, E.: Effect of glucagon and glomerulopressin on the renal function of the dog. Horm. Metab. Res. *11:* 275–279 (1979b).
Ussing, H.H.: Volume regulation and basolateral co-transport of sodium, potassium, and chloride ions in frog skin epithelium. Pflügers Arch. *405:* suppl. 1, pp S2–S7 (1985).

Ussing, H. H.: Epithelial cell volume regulation illustrated by experiments in frog skin. Renal Physiol. *9:* 38–46 (1986).
Ussing, H. H.: Volume regulation in frog skin epithelium. Comp. Physiol. *4:* 87–113 (1989).
Ussing, H. H.: Volume regulation of frog skin epithelium. Comp. Physiol. *4:* 87–113 (1990).
Vislie, T.: Cell volume regulation in fish heart ventricles with special reference to taurine. Compar. Biochem. Physiol. *76A:* 507–514 (1983).
Völkl, H.; Lang, F.: Electrophysiology of cell volume regulation in proximal tubules of the mouse kidney. Pflügers Arch. *411:* 514–519 (1988a).
Völkl, H.; Lang, F.: Ionic requirement for regulatory cell volume decrease in renal straight proximal tubules. Pflügers Arch. *412:* 1–6 (1988b).
Völkl, H.; Paulmichl, M.; Lang, F.: Cell volume regulation in renal cortical cells. Renal Physiol. Biochem. *11:* 158–173 (1988).
Vom Dahl, S.; Hallbrucker, C.; Lang, F.; Häussinger, D.: Role of eicosanoids, inositol phosphates and extracellular Ca^{++} in cell volume regulation of rat liver. Eur. J. Biochem. *198:* 73–83 (1991).
Weiss, H.; Lang, F.: Ion channels activated by swelling of Madin Darby canine kidney (MDCK)-cells. J. Membr. Biol. *126:* 109–114 (1992).
Welling, P. A.; Linshaw, M. A.; Sullivan, L. P.: Effect of barium on cell volume regulation in rabbit proximal straight tubules. Am. J. Physiol. *249:* F20–F27 (1985).
Welling, P. A.; O'Neill, R. G.: Cell swelling activates basolateral membrane Cl and K conductances in rabbit proximal tubule. Am. J. Physiol. *258:* F951–F962 (1990).
Wettstein, M.; Vom Dahl, S.; Lang, F.; Gerok, W.; Häussinger, D.: Cell volume regulatory responses of isolated perfused rat liver. The effect of amino acids. Biol. Chem. Hoppe-Seyler *371:* 493–501 (1990).
Wiener, H.; Turnheim, K.: Calcium-activated potassium channels in basolateral membranes of colon epithelial cells, reconstitution and functional properties. Wien. klin. Wschr. *26:* 622–628 (1990).
Yamauchi, A.; Kwon, H. M.; Uchida, S.; Preston, A. S.; Handler, J. S.: Myo-inositol and betaine transporters regulated by tonicity are basolateral in MDCK cells. Am. J. Physiol. *261:* F197–F202 (1991).
Yantorno, R. E.; Coca-Prados, M.; Krupin, T.; Civan, M. M.: Volume regulation of cultured transformed, non-pigmented epithelial cells from human ciliary body. Exp. Eye Res. *49:* 423–437 (1989).

Renal Physiol Biochem 1993;16:66–78

Rolf K. H. Kinne
Ralf-Peter Czekay
Julia M. Grunewald
Frank C. Mooren
Evamaria Kinne-Saffran

Max-Planck-Institut für Systemphysiologie, Dortmund, FRG

Hypotonicity-Evoked Release of Organic Osmolytes from Distal Renal Cells: Systems, Signals, and Sidedness

Key Words
Organic osmolytes
Sorbitol
Intracellular Ca^{2+}
Transport proteins
Volume regulation
Collecting duct
Membrane recycling

Abstract
After a detailed description of early cellular, membrane and intracellular events in rat renal medullary collecting duct cells when exposed to hypotonicity, a synopsis on organic osmolyte transport properties, possible trigger mechanisms, and the cellular location of transport pathways is given. From the data currently available on renal and nonrenal cells, it is concluded that hypotonicity-evoked efflux of all organic osmolytes appears to be mediated by transport proteins which share a variety of properties more typical for channels than for carriers. A large diversity seems to exist, however, for the signalling mechanisms. Such diversity allows the cells to regulate the intracellular concentration of different organic osmolytes independently of each other, giving flexibility to the spectrum of osmotic responses. The site of release also varies from cell to cell; here conservation of organic osmolytes for future reuptake or further metabolism appears to be the major determinant.

Introduction

It is now firmly established that organic osmolytes play an important role in the regulation of volume in cells as diverse as glial cells, retinal cells, hepatocytes, red blood cells, and renal cells [1–14]. For the latter in vivo and in vitro studies have identified sorbitol, myoinositol, taurine, glycerophosphorylcholine, and betaine as the major organic osmolytes [15–23]. The osmotic regulation of their intracellular concentration can involve modulation of synthesis or degradation, changes in cellular uptake or alterations of cellular release. These various mechanisms are often used in combination with different

Rolf K. H. Kinne
Max-Planck-Institut für molekulare Physiologie
Rheinlanddamm 201
D-W-4600 Dortmund (FRG)

1011–6524/93/
0162–0066 $2.75/0

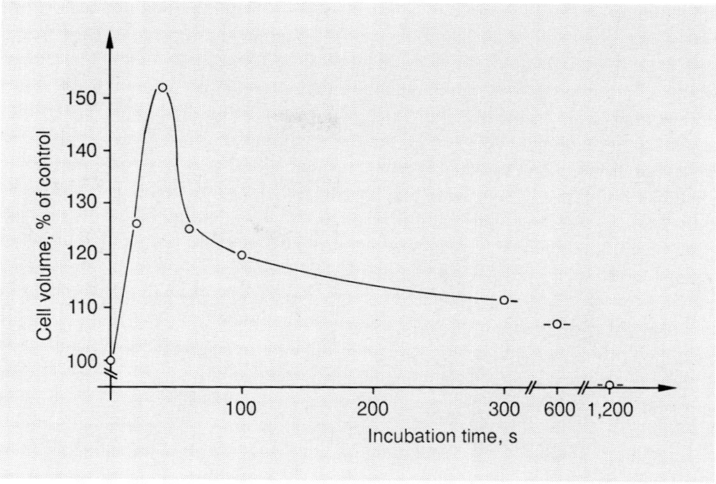

Fig. 1. Time course of volume changes in isolated rat renal IMCD cells during exposure to hypo-osmotic solutions. Cells were isolated according to Stokes et al. [35] at 600 mosm/l and suspended at time zero in a medium of 300 mosm/l. The osmolality was changed by varying the sodium chloride concentration [Data are taken from 36, 37, with kind permission].

time courses, involving different trigger mechanisms, and depending on the osmotic conditions the cell is exposed to [24–35].

This review concentrates on the rapid release of organic osmolytes observed after lowering the extracellular osmolarity and delineates the similarities and dissimilarities between the hypotonicity-induced fluxes of organic osmolytes in various cells.

Response of Rat Renal Inner Medullary Collecting Duct Cells on Exposure to Hypotonicity

Cell Volume

As shown in figure 1, exposure of inner medullary collecting duct (IMCD) cells isolated at 600 mosm/l to a medium made hypotonic by removal of NaCl leads to a very rapid transient increase in intracellular volume, followed by a regulatory volume decrease (RVD). Within the accuracy of the time resolution of the volume measurement, the peak of cell swelling seems to be reached around 40 s after exposure of the cells to hypotonicity, backregulation of the cell volume is complete after 15 min [36, 37].

Intracellular Inorganic Osmolytes

If the time course of changes of intracellular potassium, sodium, and chloride under the same experimental conditions is considered (see table 1), the total intracellular osmolality contributed by these inorganic electrolytes increases rather than decreases during RVD, suggesting that other osmolytes must leave the cells during this time period to reestablish osmotic equilibrium [37–40].

Sorbitol Flux

It has been noted previously by several authors [24, 26, 31, 41] that the sorbitol content of IMCD cells is drastically decreased during prolonged exposure to hypotonic media by an increase in plasma membrane permeability to this polyol. The actual time course of changes in apparent sorbitol permeability, as calculated from the fluxes and the transmembrane gradients is depicted in figure 2. Within 60 s the sorbitol permeability increases 45-fold and then declines gradually to the control value which is reached between 10 and 20 min of hypotonic exposure. Thus, rapid efflux of sorbitol (and probably also other organic osmolytes) can explain the apparently paradoxical

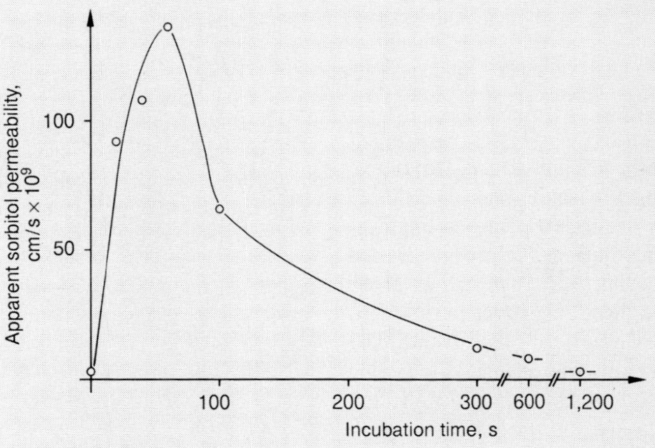

Fig. 2. Time course of changes in apparent sorbitol permeability during exposure of isolated rat renal IMCD cells to hypo-osmotic solutions [Data are taken from 36, with kind permission].

Table 1. Changes of inorganic osmolytes during exposure of rat renal IMCD cells to hypo-osmotic solutions: Sum of intracellular potassium, sodium and chloride concentration

Time min	Cells kept at 600 mosm	Cells exposed to 300 mosm/l
0	260±13	
1	280±24	159±8
2	286±10	186±10
3	272±16	190±18
4	270±3	190±18
5	290±9	206±16

Data taken from Grunewald [37] with kind permission.

behavior of cell volume and intracellular inorganic electrolyte content.

It is also noteworthy that the changes in cell volume and sorbitol permeability can be dissociated on several scales. The peak of cell swelling occurs about 20 s earlier than the peak in sorbitol permeability, the change in sorbitol permeability is much more pronounced than the volume change, and the drop in sorbitol permeability is faster than RVD, suggesting that membrane stretching and membrane sorbitol permeability are not directly proportional to each other. Thus, an additional trigger mechanism must exist.

The Role of Intracellular Calcium

In 1990 Bevan et al. [42] reported that hypotonicity-evoked sorbitol release from IMCD cells was markedly decreased when calcium was absent from the incubation medium. In addition, it could be demonstrated that ionomycin added to cells suspended in isotonic incubation media doubled the sorbitol efflux in the presence of calcium but not in its absence. Under these experimental conditions no swelling of the IMCD cells was observed, thus again a dissociation between increased sorbitol permeability and membrane stretching could be found. Furthermore, it was observed that trifluoperazine almost completely blocked the hypotonicity-evoked sorbitol efflux. Taken together, these experiments suggested that an increase in intracellular calcium might be a signal in the chain of events leading to the osmotic regulation of plasma membrane permeability. It should be noted that in IMCD cells release of glycero-

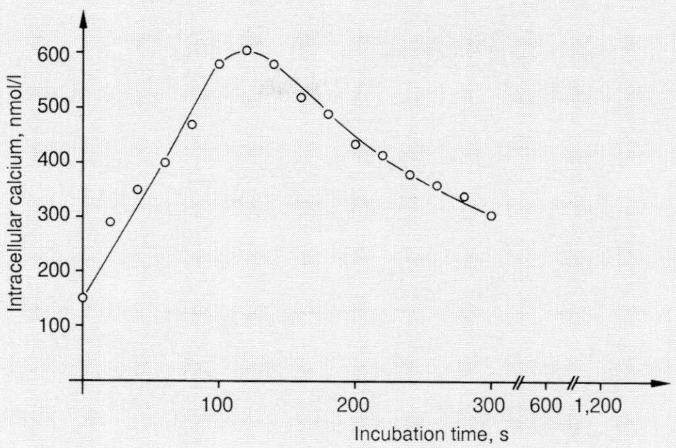

Fig. 3. Time course of changes in intracellular calcium during exposure of rat renal IMCD cells in primary culture to hypo-osmotic solution. For technical reasons the decrease of osmolality in this experimental setup takes about 45 s, therefore a direct comparison between this time course and those given in figures 1 and 2 is not possible. In addition, the osmolality of the incubation medium was changed by decreasing the sucrose content [Data redrawn from 44, with kind permission].

phosphorylcholine was not altered by changes in calcium concentration or by addition of ionomycin or trifluoperazine [43], indicating a different regulation of this transport pathway.

Subsequently, as shown in fig. 3, it was found that intracellular calcium, indeed, undergoes rapid changes during the exposure of IMCD cells to hypotonicity. During the first minute intracellular calcium increases rapidly about 4-fold and then decreases again rather quickly and approaches a plateau phase after 5 min. After reexposure to isotonicity, intracellular calcium returns immediately to control levels. These calcium transients show the same osmotic thresholds as sorbitol release and there is an identical inhibition profile with regard to the effect of calcium channel blockers on calcium influx and sorbitol efflux. All these experiments suggest a close link between intracellular calcium and sorbitol permeability [44].

Membrane Recycling

In attempting to identify the mechanism by which changes in intracellular calcium might modulate the sorbitol permeability of the plasma membrane, it became evident that calcium-dependent kinases (protein kinase C) are probably not directly involved in this process since neither inhibitors of the kinase, such as H7, nor stimulators, such as phorbolesters and diacylglycerol, affected sorbitol release before or after exposure to hypotonicity. Other kinases also seem to be excluded since cAMP and cGMP and their membrane-permeant congeners were also ineffective [42].

The observations that during the hypotonicity-evoked calcium influx a rapid and transient disintegration of the submembranal actin network occurred and that cytochalasin D pretreatment of IMCD cells attenuated the hypotonicity-evoked sorbitol release [36] finally led to the hypothesis that cytoskeleton-linked membrane recycling processes might be involved in regulating the sorbitol permeability of the plasma membrane. Such recycling processes have been invoked for example in collecting duct cells with regard to the regulation of the water permeability of the luminal membrane [45, 46].

A scheme of a membrane recycling process is presented in figure 4. The increase in intracellular calcium is postulated to allow access of sorbitol transporter-carrying aggrego-

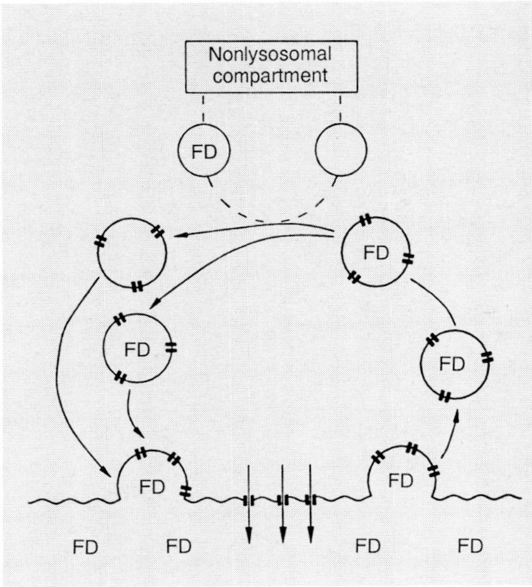

Fig. 4. Scheme of hypotonicity-induced membrane recycling assumed to be involved in the regulation of sorbitol permeability. The pairs of short parallel bars represent sorbitol transporters [taken from 36, with kind permission].

phores (or reserve vesicles) and fusion of these aggregophores with the plasma membrane. The subsequent decline in intracellular calcium would initiate the retrieval of transporter-rich membrane areas and finally, when calcium levels reach control levels, sorbitol permeability would also be normalized. Evidence for the operation of such a mechanism was provided from a variety of experiments, two of them will be discussed in more detail. First it was demonstrated that during RVD IMCD cells take up fluorescein-labeled dextran (molecular weight 74,000 daltons) and that this uptake has a time course similar to the decrease in plasma membrane sorbitol permeability after its initial augmentation. Representative experiments are shown in figure 5. Using fluorescent dextran (FD) as a fluid marker, after 100 s – but not earlier – a labeling of IMCD cells just below the plasma membrane is observed. This labeling increases strongly during the following incubation period. At the same time sorbitol permeability of the plasma membrane is reduced from 45 times the normal value to 2 times the control. When such FD-labeled IMCD cells are subjected to a second hypotonic shock, the release of FD from the cells and the increase in sorbitol release show initially a very similar time course and, as depicted in figure 6, are closely related under different experimental maneuvers. These observations taken together are in agreement with the above proposed model of membrane recycling [36, 47, 48].

Sidedness of Sorbitol Release

The labeling procedure described above can also be used to define the direction of sorbitol release from the IMCD cells. In longitudinal optical sections of IMCD cells obtained by confocal laser scanning microscopy after exposure to hypotonicity induced labeling could only be observed at the basal-lateral cell side (see fig. 7). Similar results were obtained in electron-microscopic investigations using colloidal iron as a marker for endocytic processes [36]. In the same figure labeling of the apical cell pole is demonstrated, which had been induced by transient exposure of the cells to antidiuretic hormone in the presence of dextran labeled with Texas Red. This labeling is due to retrieval of water channel-containing aggregophores from the luminal membrane [45, 47, 49].

The Sorbitol Transporter in IMCD Cells

The molecular properties of the sorbitol transporter have been studied thus far only at the cellular level. The transporter seems to be strongly rectified since in IMCD cells exposed to hypotonic medium containing radioactively labeled sorbitol strong sorbitol efflux but no uptake of labeled sorbitol could be observed. The transporter seems to be relatively specif-

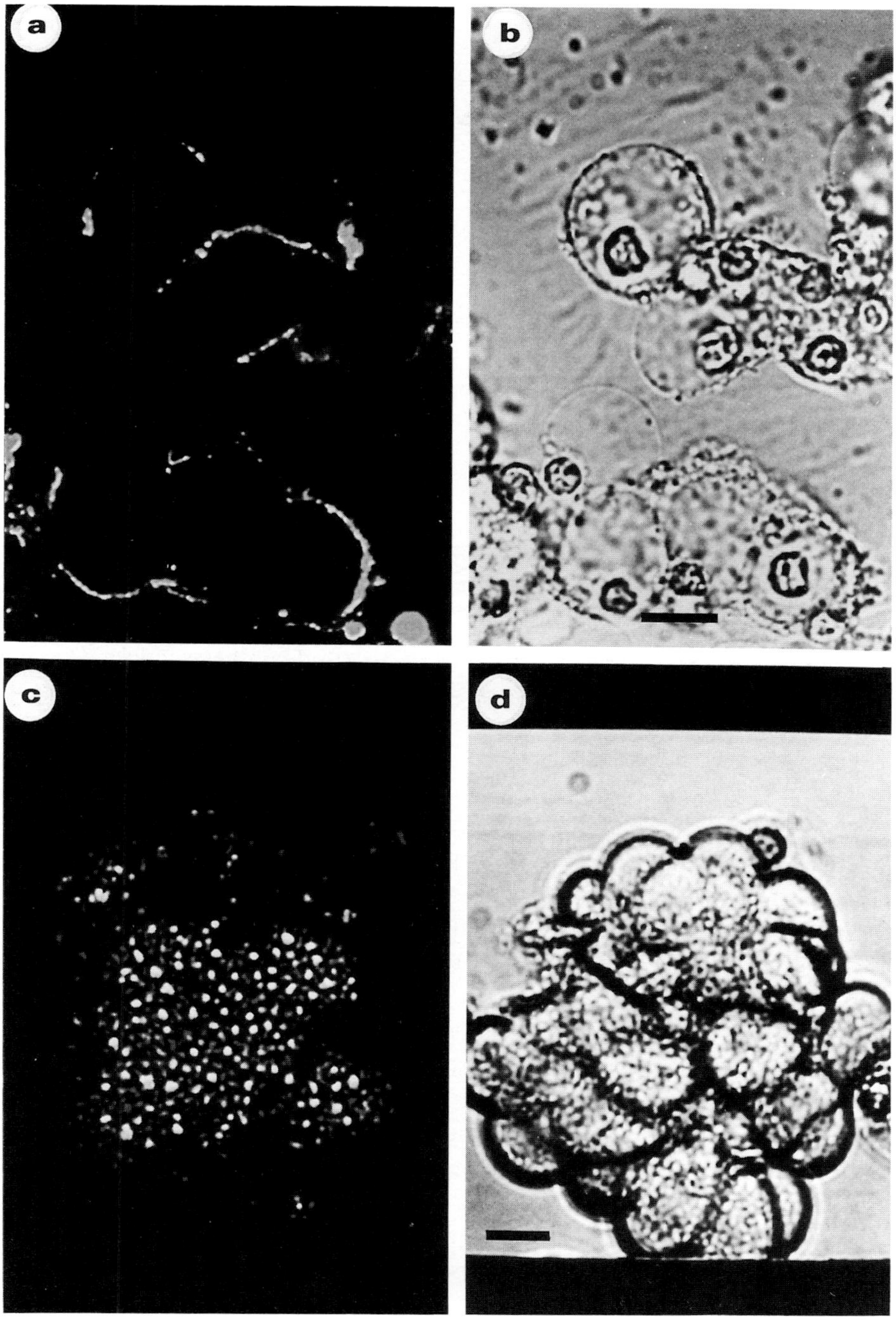

Fig. 5. Time course of FD uptake into rat renal IMCD cells during exposure to hypotonic medium. **a**, **b** Uptake after 100 s. **c**, **d** Uptake after 5 min. Cofocal laser scanning microscopy image [from 36, with kind permission]. Bar represents 7 μm.

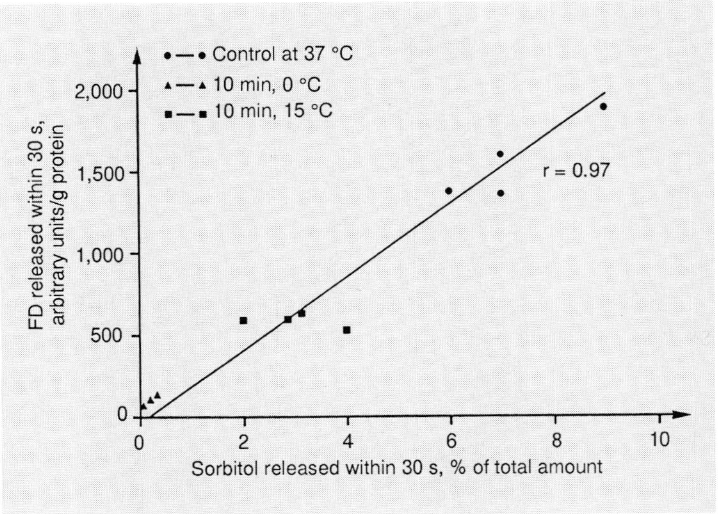

Fig. 6. Correlation between FD release and increase in sorbitol permeability at different temperatures after exposure of FD-labeled IMCD cells to a second hypotonic shock [from 36, with kind permission].

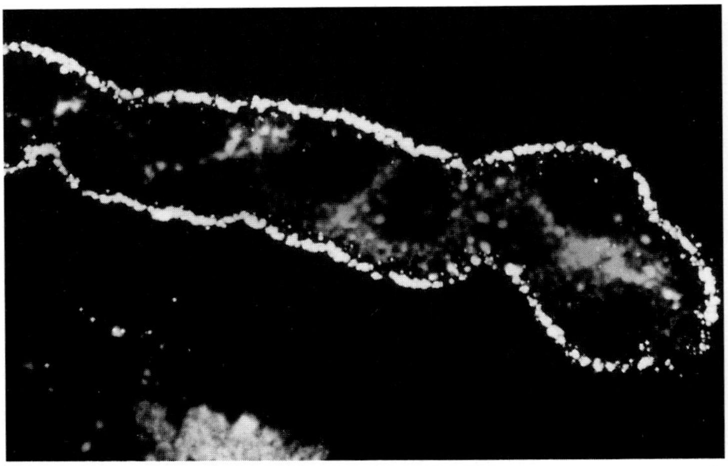

Fig. 7. Sidedness of hypotonicity-induced labeling of rat renal IMCD cells with FD (white vesicles) as contracted to membrane retrieval induced by transient exposure of the cells to antidiuretic hormone (grey areas). Confocal laser scanning microscopy image [from 36, with kind permission].

ic: *D*-glucose is not released by osmotic shock and myoinositol release shows a different time course of release [26, 43]. In addition, changing sorbitol concentrations inside the cells by using different glucose concentrations in the medium failed to reveal a saturability of the efflux pathway.

There are, however, several inhibitors of efflux. Decrease in temperature reduces sorbitol efflux not only in hypotonic but also in isotonic media, suggesting an effect of membrane fluidity on the transport rate [26]. Interestingly enough a number of inhibitors of potassium or chloride channels, although at high concentrations, also reduces sorbitol efflux from IMCD cells (see table 2). These include quinidine, SITS and NPPB. Finally there is a distinct inhibitory effect of PCMBS, a sulfhydryl reagent on sorbitol efflux, also in nonhypotonically treated cells, indicating the proteinous nature of the carrier [Bevan et al., unpubl. data].

Table 2. Nature of hypotonicity-evoked organic osmolyte transport systems

Osmolyte	Cells	Kinetic properties	Inhibitors	Stimulators (at isotonicity)	References
Taurine	MDCK cells	no saturation, temperature-independent, peak of activation after 10 min	quinidine (0.2 mM = 26% inhibition) DIDS (0.1 mM = 49% inhibition)		32
	astrocytes	no saturation, temperature-independent, strictly gradient-dependent, peak of activation after 1 min	quinidine (0.2 mM = 47% inhibition) DIDS (0.2 mM = 31% inhibition) 9-AC (1 mM = 68% inhibition) PCMBS (10^{-5} M ~50% inhibition)		1, 3, 4
Sorbitol	GRB-PAP1 cells (rabbit papillary epithelium)	no saturation, maximal activation within 0.5 min, temperature-sensitive, no competition by other polyols	quinidine (1 mM = 73% inhibition)		50
	rat renal IMCD cells	rectifying activation, peak of activation after 1 min, temperature-sensitive	quinidine (1 mM = 50% inhibition) trifluoperazine (20 µM = 60% inhibition) Ca channel blocker (Ba^{2+} 5 mM ~90% inhibition), Ca-free solution (80% inhibition), cytochalasin D (50 µM = 80% inhibition) SITS (1 mM = 90% inhibition) NPPB (1 mM –30% inhibition)	increase in intracellular Ca; (A23187 + Ca^{2+})	26, 36, 37, 42, 47, 48
	PAP-HT25 membrane vesicles	temperature-dependent efflux, sorbitol efflux, faster than raffinose efflux, activated by exposure of cells to hypotonicity	quinidine (1 mM ~50% inhibition)		50, 51
	PAP-HT25 cells	fast transient increase in efflux, specificity: sorbitol > mannitol > inositol	ETYA (0.1 mM = 82% inhibition) ketoconazole (0.1 mM = 91% inhibition)	mellitin (phospholipase A_2 activation, 1 µM = ~40-fold)	25, 50
Betaine	PAP-HT25 cells		ETYA (0.1 mM ~90% inhibition) ketoconazole (0.1 mM ~90% inhibition)		25
Myoinositol	PAP-HT25 cells		ETYA (0.1 mM ~90% inhibtion) ketoconazole (0.1 mM ~90% inhibition)		25

DIDS = 4,4′-Diisothiocyanostilbene-2,2′-disulfonic acid; ETYA = eicosatetraynoic acid; NPPB = 5-nitro-2-(3-phenylpropyl-amino)-benzoate; PCBMS = *p*-chloromercurybenzene-sulfonate; SITS = 4-acetamido-4′-isothiocyanostilbene-2,2-′-disulfonic acid.

Comparison between Different Cells and Different Osmolytes

Properties of Hypotonicity-Invoked Osmolyte Release (Systems)

In table 2 the properties of hypotonicity-induced efflux of taurine, sorbitol, glycerophosphorylcholine, betaine, and myoinositol are compiled that are observed in a variety of renal and nonrenal cells.

In considering this synopsis, the first striking observation is the widespread occurrence of organic osmolytes and their regulation by hypotonicity. The selection presented in table 2 represents, however, only a small part of the broad spectrum of organisms where organic osmolytes have been found [12]. It is also obvious that there are strong similarities in the kinetic properties of the efflux pathways for the different osmolytes. All systems studied thus far exhibit no saturability even at very high substrate concentrations (up to hundreds of mmol/l) and fluxes are in most cases strictly dependent on transmembrane concentration differences. Another similarity is the inhibition of the majority of these systems by quinidine and stilbene derivatives. Some of the systems are also inhibited by high concentrations of lipophilic aromatic inhibitors of anion channels.

Taking all these properties together, several authors suggested that the hypotonicity-evoked efflux pathways might represent channel-like proteins rather than carrier proteins [50–52]. Evidence for this hypothesis is based mainly on the general lack of saturability and the relatively low temperature dependence in some systems. The effect of the various channel blockers is thereby explained by a perturbation of the lipids surrounding the transport protein rather than by specific interactions between the inhibitors and the protein. Despite this possibility a word of caution is necessary. In most inhibitor studies it cannot be discerned whether the transport system itself or the events triggering the increased permeability have been affected. Some of the above-discussed properties have, however, been described in isolated membrane vesicles [51]. Thus, more defined studies at the membrane and at the molecular level are necessary to prove or disprove the hypothesis on the channel-like structure of organic osmolyte pathways.

Such channel-like properties of transporters for organic molecules have already been described recently for the glutamate transporter in renal brush border membranes and in mitochondria. In the former, even transition between a carrier-like operation and a channel-like operation can be induced by changes in pH [53].

Mechanisms of Activation (Signals)

Table 2 also compiles the information currently available on potential modes of activation of the efflux mechanisms. A frequently observed characteristic is the fast response to cell swelling and the relatively rapid reversibility of the response. Therefore, membrane stretching has to be taken into account as one possible mechanism of activation, similar to the activation of calcium channels by changes in membrane surface tension [54]. Such a direct coupling remains, however, to be demonstrated and cannot be considered as the sole mechanism since the different osmolytes show different osmotic thresholds. With regard to intracellular signals intracellular calcium seems to be involved in the regulation of sorbitol permeability of rat renal IMCD cells and in Madin-Darby canine kidney (MDCK) cells. In rabbit papillary epithelial cell culture and rabbit inner medullary cells the hypo-osmotic response is, however, essentially calcium-independent [25, 51, 55]. In the rabbit papillary epithelial cells instead yet unidentified metabolites of the arachidonic acid pathway have been proposed to be involved in intracellular signalling [25]. For taurine release from skate erythrocytes the inositol triphosphate cascade seems to be important [56]. Thus, the signals for activation of a particular osmolyte efflux pathway appear to vary not only from species to species but are also different for various organic osmolytes. Unique signalling pathways seem to be physiologically reasonable since they allow the cells to adjust their response to the degree of osmotic challenge and to establish the optimum balance between the cell protective action exerted by certain organic osmolytes, such as methylamines [12, 57], and their osmotic activity.

Table 3. Sidedness of organic osmolyte release in renal cells

Cell type	Organic osmolyte	Cell side	References
MDCK cells (on membrane filters)	taurine	apical	34; Sanchez-Oléa, unpubl.
	betaine	basolateral	66
	myoinositol	basolateral	66
Papillary cells in culture			
on membrane filters	sorbitol	apical	7, 24, 50
	myoinositol	apical	27
on plastic	sorbitol	apical?	24
	GPC	apical?	7
	betaine	apical?	27
IMCD cells (freshly isolated and on membrane filters)	sorbitol	basolateral	36, 37

The proposed modes of activation range from the hypothesis of membrane recycling [36, 47, 48] or a stretch activation [54, 58–65] to a direct modification of transporters that can still be demonstrated in vitro after the isolation of plasma membranes from rabbit papillary epithelium cell cultures [51]. The nature of modification of the transport systems is still unknown; phosphorylation reactions mediated by cAMP, cGMP, or calcium-activated kinases seem unlikely in view of the lack of effect of cAMP and cGMP on sorbitol fluxes both in rat and rabbit papillary cells.

Sidedness of Release

In table 3 results on investigations addressing the question of sidedness of release are compiled. In analyzing these data the degree of differentiation of the epithelial cells investigated has to be considered. In highly polarized and differentiated MDCK cells taurine is released across the apical membrane, whereas betaine and myoinositol leave the cell across the basal-lateral membrane [66]. The luminal release of taurine would coincide with the general direction of taurine transport in renal epithelia where secretion of this end-product of metabolism prevails [67]. The basal-lateral release of betaine and myoinositol might be related to the presence of sodium cotransport systems for these two organic osmolytes in the contraluminal membrane [66].

Thus, locally a reservoir of organic osmolytes might be generated that can be used to regain intracellular osmolytes rather quickly when the extracellular sodium and chloride increases after the diuretic phase. The parallel presence of leak pathways and uptake systems in the same membrane is not necessarily counterproductive. During hypotonic shock strong electrogenic sodium cotransport systems might be reduced in their activity by changes in driving forces and thereby reuptake could be minimized.

In freshly isolated IMCD cells and in IMCD cells cultured on a permeable filter support sorbitol release occurs at the contraluminal cell side [36; Grunewald, pers. communication]. This can be concluded indirectly from the labeling studies presented above and was demonstrated directly by measuring sorbitol fluxes. In the inner medulla this direction of release might be a mechanism to preserve the carbohydrate for further intramedullary metabolism. In this context the observation is important that during the purification of IMCD cells from rat kidney the aldose reductase activity (catalyzing sorbitol formation from *D*-glucose) in the cells continuously increases, whereas the activity of the sorbitol dehydrogenase (catalyzing the oxidation of sorbitol to fructose) decreases [68]. This result suggests that renal medullary cells (other than IMCD cells) are capable of further metabolizing sorbitol. Thereby the carbon skeleton of sorbitol could be metabolically preserved.

Epithelial cells grown on plastic substratum are generally not as differentiated as those grown on permeable filters or their counterpart in vivo. This lower degree of differentiation is accompanied by 'missorting' of at least some membrane components [69]. In such systems conclusions on cellular location of efflux pathways are, therefore, not unequivocal. The degree of confluency and the tightness of the intercellular junctions can also affect the results. Therefore, differences observed in various cell types might be apparent and not real. Further experiments on well-defined systems are therefore necessary to get more solid information on the sidedness of release of the various osmolytes in different cell types.

Concluding Remarks

From the brief summary presented above it is obvious that there exist still large gaps in our knowledge on systems, signals and sidedness with regard to the hypotonically evoked release of organic osmolytes from renal and other cells. This field of investigation poses, however, several interesting basic questions in membrane transport, intracellular signalling and epithelial cell biology. Answering these questions will, therefore, not only lead to a better understanding of renal medullary cell physiology and pathophysiology but also to deeper insights into cell biology in general.

Acknowledgements

The collaborative efforts of all my colleagues to compile this review is gratefully acknowledged. Without the skill and persistence of D. Mägdefessel this manuscript would never have been completed.

Remembering the hospitality extended to us in Naples by Natale de Santo and Giovambattista Capasso also provided a strong positive driving force.

References

1 Schousboe A, Sánchez Olea R, Morán J, Pasantes-Morales H: Hyposmolarity-induced taurine release in cerebellar granule cells is associated with diffusion and not with high-affinity transport. J Neurosci Res 1991;30:661–665.
2 Wiesinger H, Thiess U, Hamprecht B: Sorbitol pathway activity and utilization of polyols in astroglia-rich primary cultures. Glia 1990;3: 277–282.
3 Morán J, Hurtado S, Pasantes-Morales H: Similar properties of taurine release induced by potassium and hyposmolarity in the rat retina. Exp Eye Res 1991;53:347–352.
4 Sánchez-Olea R, Morán J, Pasantes-Morales H: Changes in taurine transport evoked by hyperosmolarity in cultured astrocytes. J Neurosci Res 1992;32:86–92.
5 Wiesinger H: *myo*-Inositol transport in mouse astroglia-rich primary culture. J Neurochem 1991;56: 1698–1704.
6 Pasantes-Morales H, Morán J, Sánchez Olea R: Volume regulatory fluxes in glial and renal cells. Adv Exp Med Biol 1992;315:361–368.
7 Garcia-Perez A, Burg MB: Renal medullary organic osmolytes. Physiol Rev 1991;71:1081–1115.
8 Forster RP, Goldstein L: Intracellular osmoregulatory role of amino acids and urea in marine elasmobranchs. Am J Physiol 1976;230: 925–931.

9 Gilles R: Comparative aspects of cell osmoregulation and volume control. Renal Physiol Biochem 1988;11:277–288.
10 Robertson JD: Chemical composition of the body fluids and muscle of the hagfish *Myxine glutinosa* and the rabbit-fish *Chimaera monstrosa*. J Zool 1976;178:261–277.
11 Wolff SD, Balaban RS: Regulation of the predominant renal medullary organic solutes in vivo. Annu Rev Physiol 1990;52:727–746.
12 Yancey PH, Clark ME, Hand SC, Bowlus RD, Somero GN: Living with water stress: Evolution of osmolyte systems. Science 1982;217: 1214–1222.
13 Boyd TA, Cha C-J, Forster RP, Goldstein L: Free amino acids in tissues of the skate *Raja erinacea* and the stingray *Dasyatis sabina:* Effects of environmental dilution. J Exp Zool 1977;199:435–442.
14 Boyer JL, Graf J, Meier PJ: Hepatic transport systems regulating pH_i, cell volume, and bile secretion. Annu Rev Physiol 1992;54:415–438.
15 Bagnasco SM, Balaban RS, Fales HM, Yang Y-M, Burg MB: Predominant osmotically active organic solutes in rat and rabbit renal medullas. J Biol Chem 1986;261: 5872–5877.
16 Balaban RS, Burg MB: Osmotically active organic solutes in the renal inner medulla. Kidney Int 1987;31: 562–564.
17 Beck FX, Dörge A, Thurau K, Guder WG: Cell osmoregulation in their countercurrent system of the renal medulla: The role of organic osmolytes. Comp Physiol 1990;4: 132–158.
18 Nakanishi T, Balaban RB, Burg MB: Survey of osmolytes in renal cell lines. Am J Physiol 1988;255: C181–C191.
19 Schimassek H, Kohl D, Bücher T: Glycerolphosphorylcholine, die Nierensubstanz 'Ma-Mark' von Ullrich. Biochem Z 1959;331:87–97.
20 Ullrich KJ, Pehling G: Über das Vorkommen von Phosphorverbindungen in verschiedenen Nierenabschnitten und Änderungen ihrer Konzentration in Abhängigkeit vom Diuresezustand. Pflügers Arch 1956;262:551–561.
21 Wolff SD, Eng C, Balaban RS: NMR studies of renal phosphate metabolites in vivo: Effects of hydration and dehydration. Am J Physiol 1988;255:F581–F589.
22 Balaban RS, Knepper MA: Nitrogen-14 nuclear magnetic resonance spectroscopy of mammalian tissues. Am J Physiol 1983;245:C439–C444.
23 Billadello JJ, Gard JK, Ackerman JJH, Gross RW: Determination of intact-tissue glycerophosphorylcholine levels by quantitative ^{31}P nuclear magnetic resonance spectroscopy and correlation with spectrophotometric quantification. Anal Biochem 1985;144:269–274.
24 Bagnasco SM, Murphy HR, Bedford JJ, Burg MB: Osmoregulation by slow changes in aldose reductase and rapid changes in sorbitol flux. Am J Physiol 1988;254:C788–C792.
25 Furlong TJ, Moriyama T, Spring KR: Activation of osmolyte efflux from cultured renal papillary epithelial cells. J Membr Biol 1991; 123:269–277.
26 Grunewald RW, Kinne RKH: Intracellular sorbitol content in isolated rat inner medullary collecting duct cells. Regulation by extracellular osmolarity. Pflügers Arch 1989; 414:178–184.
27 Nakanishi T, Turner RJ, Burg MB: Osmoregulatory changes in *myo*-inositol transport by renal cells. Proc Natl Acad Sci USA 1989;86:6002–6006.
28 Nakanishi T, Turner RJ, Burg MB: Osmoregulation of betaine transport in mammalian renal medullary cells. Am J Physiol 1990;258: F1061–F1067.
29 Nakanishi T, Uyama O, Sugita M: Osmotically regulated taurine content in rat renal innner medulla. Am J Physiol 1991;261:F957–F962.
30 Zablocki K, Miller S, Garcia-Perez A, Burg M: Accumulation of glycerophosphorylcholine (GPC) by renal cells: Osmotic regulation of GPC:choline phosphodiesterase. Proc Natl Acad Sci USA 1991;88: 7820–7824.
31 Wirthensohn G, Lefrank S, Schmolke M, Guder WG: Regulation of organic osmolyte concentrations in tubules from rat renal inner medulla. Am J Physiol 1989;256: F128–F135.
32 Uchida S, Nakanishi T, Kwon HM, Preston AS, Handler JS: Taurine behaves as an osmolyte in Madin-Darby canine kidney cells. Protection by polarized, regulated transport of taurine. J Clin Invest 1991; 88:656–662.
33 Known HM, Yamauchi A, Uchida S, Robey RB, Garcia-Perez A, Burg MB, Handler JS: Renal Na-*myo*-inositol cotransporter mRNA expression in *Xenopus* oocytes: regulation by hypertonicity. Am J Physiol 1991;260:F258–F263.
34 Bagnasco SM, Uchida S, Balaban RS, Kador P, Burg MB: Induction of aldose reductase and sorbitol in renal inner medulla cells by elevated extracellular NaCl. Proc Natl Acad Sci USA 1987;84:1718–1720.
35 Stokes JB, Grupp C, Kinne RKH: Purification of rat papillary collecting duct cells: Functional and metabolic assessment. Am J Physiol 1987;253:F251–F262.
36 Czekay R-P: Osmo- und Volumenregulation in isolierten Sammelrohrzellen der inneren Medulla der Rattenniere (IMCD). Die Rolle der Plasmamembran und des Cytoskeletts bei der Freisetzung des organischen Osmolyts Sorbitol. PhD Thesis Ruhr-Universität Bochum, 1991.
37 Grunewald JM: Volumenregulation und Ionenflüsse in isolierten Sammelrohrzellen der inneren Medulla der Rattenniere. MD Thesis Heinrich-Heine-Universität, Düsseldorf, 1992.
38 Beck F, Dörge A, Rick R, Thurau K: Intra- and extracellular element concentrations of rat renal papilla in antidiuresis. Kidney Int 1984;25: 397–403.
39 Beck F, Dörge A, Rick R, Thurau K: Osmoregulation of renal papillary cells. Pflügers Arch 1985;405: S28–S32.
40 Beck FX, Dörge A, Thurau K: Cellular osmoregulation in the renal papilla. Klin Wochenschr 1988;66: 843–848.
41 Beck FX, Dörge A, Thurau K: Cellular osmoregulation in renal medulla. Renal Physiol Biochem 1988; 11:174–186.

42 Bevan C, Theiss C, Kinne RKH: Role of Ca^{2+} in sorbitol release from rat inner medullary collecting duct (IMCD) cells under hypoosmotic stress. Biochem Biophys Res Commun 1990;170:563–568.
43 Bauernschmitt HG: Untersuchungen zu Funktion, Regulation und Metabolismus des 'organischen Osmolyts' Glycerophosphorylcholin (GPC) in papillären Sammelrohrzellen (IMCD) der Rattenniere. PhD Thesis Ruhr-Universität Bochum, 1991.
44 Mooren FCh: Untersuchungen zur Rolle des Kalziums in der Volumenregulation papillärer Sammelrohrzellen der Ratte. MD Thesis, Heinrich-Heine-Universität, Düsseldorf, 1993.
45 Hays RM: Water transport in epithelia. Comp Physiol 1990;2:1–30.
46 Verkman AS: Water channels in cell membranes. Annu Rev Physiol 1992;54:97–108.
47 Czekay R-P, Bevan C, Kinne RKH: Membrane traffic and sorbitol release during osmoregulation in isolated rat renal inner medullary collecting duct (IMCD) cells. Pflügers Arch 1991;418:R69.
48 Kinne RKH, Bauernschmitt HG, Bevan C, Czekay R-P: Membrane events in the control of organic osmolyte content: A study on isolated inner medullary collecting ducts (IMCD) cells. Abstract book IUPS Regional Meeting, Prague, 1991, No SB3.5.
49 Brown D, Weyer P, Orci L: Vasopressin stimulates endocytosis in kidney collecting duct principal cells. Eur J Cell Biol 1988;46:336–341.
50 Garty H, Furlong TJ, Ellis DE, Spring KR: Sorbitol permease: An apical membrane transporter in cultured renal papillary epithelial cells. Am J Physiol 1991;260:F650–F656.
51 Siebens AW, Spring KR: A novel sorbitol transport mechanism in cultured renal papillary epithelial cells. Am J Physiol 1989;257:F937–F946.
52 Kinne RKH: The role of organic osmolytes in osmoregulation: From bacteria to mammals. J Exp Zool 1993;265.
53 Kinne RKH: Glutamate-sodium cotransport in the kidney: An example for the plasticity of transport systems; in Petzinger E, Kinne RKH, Sies H (eds): Hepatic transport of Organic Substances. Berlin, Springer, 1898, pp 3–11.
54 Christensen C: Mediation of cell volume regulation by Ca influx through stretch-activated channels. Nature 1987;330:66–68.
55 Zaghow M: Untersuchungen zur Regulation von organischen Osmolyten in der inneren Medulla der Kaninchenniere, PhD Thesis Universität Hannover, 1991.
56 Musch MW, Goldstein L: Hypotonicity stimulates phosphatidylcholine hydrolysis and generates diacylglycerol in erythrocytes. J Biol Chem 1990;265:13055–13059.
57 Somero G: From dogfish to dogs: trimethylamines protect proteins from urea. NIPS 1986;1:9–12.
58 Bear CE: A nonselective cation channel in rat liver cells is activated by membrane stretch. Am J Physiol 1990;258:C421–C428.
59 Becks JS, Potts DJ: Cell swelling, co-transport activation and potassium conductance in isolated perfused rabbit kidney proximal tubules. J Physiol 1990;425:369–378.
60 Dube L, Parent L, Sauve R: Hypotonic shock activates a maxi K^+ channel in primary cultured proximal tubule cells. Am J Physiol 1990; 259:F348–F356.
61 Filipovic D, Sackin H: A calcium-permeable stretch-activated cation channel in renal proximal tubule. Am J Physiol 1991;260:F119–F129.
62 Taniguchi J, Guggino WB: Membrane stretch: A physiological stimulator of Ca^{2+}-activated K^+ channels in thick ascending limb. Am J Physiol 1989;257:F347–F352.
63 Ubl J, Murer H, Kolb HA: Ion channels activated by osmotic and mechanical stress in membranes of opossum kidney cells. J Membr Biol 1988;104:223–232.
64 Okada Y, Hazama A, Yuan W: Stretch- induced activation of $Ca^{(2+)}$-permeable ion channels is involved in the volume regulation of hypotonically swollen epithelial cells. Neurosci Res 1990;12:S5–S13.
65 McCarthy NA, O'Neil RG: Calcium-dependent control of volume regulation in renal proximal tubule cells. I. Swelling-activated Ca^{2+} entry and release. J Membr Biol 1991; 123:149–160.
66 Yamauchi A, Kwon HM, Uchida S, Preston AS, Handler JS: *Myo*-inositol and betaine transporters regulated by tonicity are basolateral in MDCK cells. Am J Physiol 1991; 261:F197–F202.
67 Kinne RKH: Selectivity and direction: Plasma membranes in renal transport. Am J Physiol 1991;260: F153–F162.
68 Grunewald RW, Jans AWH, Kinne RKH: Sorbitkonzentration und -metabolismus in der Nierenpapilla. Nieren Hochdruckkrankh 1989; 18:13–16.
69 Bacallo R, Fine LG: Molecular events in the organization of renal tubular epithelium: From nephrogenesis to regeneration. Am J Physiol 1989;257:F913–F924.

Renal Physiology Biochem 1993;16:79–88

H. Siebe[a]
G. Baude[b]
I. Lichtenstein[a]
D. Wang[a]
H. Bühler[a]
G.-A. Hoyer[b]
K. Hierholzer[a]

[a] Institut für Klinische Physiologie, Universitätsklinikum der Freien Universität Berlin, und
[b] Schering, Institut für Physikochemie, Berlin, BRD

Metabolism of Dexamethasone: Sites and Activity in Mammalian Tissues

Key Words
Dexamethasone
11β-Hydroxysteroid dehydrogenase
Corticosterone
Cortisol
Metabolism of corticosteroids
Intestinal tract
Kidney
Liver
Testicle

Abstract
We have used in vitro techniques to study the metabolism of dexamethasone. Tissue slices, homogenates and microsomal fractions of various mammalian organs from rats and humans have been used. We focused particularly on the question of whether or not dexamethasone (Dexa) is oxidized at the C_{11}-OH group by 11β-hydroxysteroid-dehydrogenase. High activities of this enzyme system for Dexa were localized in renal cortex and rectum. Material from both human and murine liver was ineffective. The main metabolite formed from Dexa in renal and intestinal systems was identified by different mass-spectrometric techniques including on line HPLC mass spectrometry as 11-dehydro-dexamethasone. This finding was corroborated by the observation that both corticosterone and glycyrrhetinic acid block the metabolic transformation of Dexa.

Introduction

The synthetic glucocorticosteroid (GCS) dexamethasone has gained wide acceptance both as a therapeutic as well as a diagnostic tool. It specifically binds to type II corticosteroid (CS) receptors, exerts many GCS functions and effectively depresses the hypothalamic-pituitary axis [1–4].

Dexamethasone (Dexa) is fluorinated at C_9 and it is generally assumed that this configuration prevents oxidative metabolic transformation at C_{11} [5, 6]. However, a survey of the literature reveals only insufficient evidence for this assumption or even provisional evidence against it [7, 8]. While it has been documented that Dexa can be metabolized in mammalian organisms neither the nature of

K. Hierholzer
Institut für Klinische Physiologie
Universitätsklinikum der Freien
Universität Berlin, Hindenburgdamm 30
D-W-1000 Berlin 45 (FRG)

1011–6524/93/
0162–0079 $2.75/0

metabolites nor the site of metabolic transformation has unequivocally been defined.

In view of the importance of the synthetic CS we have therefore attempted to study the possibility of metabolic transformation of Dexa in various mammalian tissues. We particularly address the question of a possible transformation of Dexa at C_{11} by the enzyme system 11β-hydroxysteroid-dehydrogenase (11β-HSD) (EC 1.1.1.146). The in vitro metabolism of Dexa will be compared with that of endogenous GCS, such as corticosterone (B) in rat preparations and cortisol (F) in human preparations. Direct mass-spectrometric evidence will be presented indicating that the main metabolite formed under the conditions chosen here is 11-dehydro-dexamethasone.

Methods

Biological Systems and General Techniques

Incubation techniques in vitro were performed as previously described [9, 10]. Human kidney and liver samples were obtained from surgically removed material (courtesy of the Departments of Urology + Surgery). Rat tissues (kidney, liver, testicle, intestinal tract) were excised from male Sprague-Dawley rats (Versuchstierzucht Hannover) immediately after decapitation: (a) thin slices were cut with a razor blade (~1 mm thick), (b) homogenates from various tissues were prepared with a Potter-Elvehjem homogenizer and (c) microsomes from kidneys, liver and testicles were prepared according to a modified technique of Remmer et al. [11] with glucose-6-phosphatase as marker enzyme [12].

Slices, homogenates and microsomal fractions were incubated in gassed Kh solution, or 10 μ*M* HEPES, pH 8.0, respectively, under conditions listed in tables 1–3. Homogenates and microsomal preparations were incubated without or with the addition of cosubstrates (see tables 1–3, fig. 2). In several experiments glycyrrhetinic acid (gly.ac.) was added to the incubation medium in order to specifically block 11β-HSD [13–16]. In vitro incubation was stopped after 30–60 min with ice-cold citric acid and analyzed using RP-HPLC [17]. The following hormones were used: (1) B+^{3}H-B, (2) Dexa+^{3}H-Dexa, (3) F+^{3}H-F, and furthermore the respective labelled and nonlabelled 11-dehydro (11-DH)-metabolites. Sources were New England Nuclear and Amersham Buchler; ^{3}H-DH-Dexa was prepared from ^{3}H-Dexa in our laboratory. Consubstrates (NAD$^+$/H and NADP$^+$/H) were obtained from Boehringer (Mannheim), gly.ac., from Sigma Chemicals.

Table 1. Conversion of Dexa, B and F by tissue slices

	Dexa		B	
Rat tissue				
Kidney cortex	7.1±0.4	(21)	50.1±2.5	(8)
Liver	0.4±0.1	(8)	6.3±0.5	(6)
Testicle	0.1±0.2	(12)	47.0±4.7	(6)
Duodenum	1.1±0.4	(5)	29.1±6.2	(6)
Cacum	9.0±0.7	(6)	71.9±0.9	(6)
Rectum	10.0±2.6	(22)	64.0±2.3	(12)
	Dexa		**F**	
Human tissue, (hormones 10^{-6} M)				
Kidney cortex	8.9±1.9	(6)	35.7±3.3	(6)

% conversion (means ± SE) (100% = 10^{-12} mol/100 mg tissue weight · 60 min when incubated at 10^{-9} *M* hormone concentration); conditions: parallel experiments with Dexa and B, 100 mg tissue/ml incubate (KH + substrate), 37 °C 60 min, hormones 10^{-9} *M*. Figures in parentheses indicate number.

Table 2. Conversion of the respective 11-DH-metabolities of Dexa, B and F by tissue slices

	11-DH-Dexa		11-DH-B	
Rat tissue				
Kidney cortex	42.5±2.6	(6)	31.3	(2)
	11-DH-Dexa		**11-DH-F**	
Human tissue				
Kidney cortex	61.9±2.9	(6)	1.0±0.1	(6)

For further information, see footnote to table 1.

Table 3. Conversion of Dexa, B and 11-DH-B by homogenates of rat kidney and testicle

Oxidase	Dexa				B			
	Protein µg	no cosubstrate	$+NADP^+$	$+NAD^+$	Protein µg	no cosubstrate	$+NADP^+$	$+NAD^+$
Rat kidney	200	–0.8±0.3	6.7±0.6	32.6±1.8	100	32.9±0.8	61.7±4.0	82.7±1.6
Rat testicle	200	–0.5±0.1	–0.4±0.1	–0.2±0.2	100	49.6±0.6	64.0±1.1	48.7±1.0

% conversion (means ± SE) (100% = 10^{-12} mol/protein incubated 30 min, conditions: parallel experiments with homogenates incubated in 10 m*M* HEPES pH 8.0, +/– cosubstrate ($NADP^+$/H and NAD^+/H, 10^{-3} *M*), 37°C 30 min, hormones 10^{-9} *M*, n = 6.

Analytical Techniques

Chromatographic Techniques. After the addition of citric acid the incubation vials were centrifuged and the supernatant was transferred into our isocratic RP-HPLC system. UV absorbance and radioactivity were measured on-line as previously described [9, 10] and peak areas were calculated. The hormones under study and their metabolites could be separated completely at appropriate elution conditions.

Mass-Spectrometric Techniques. Mass spectra were obtained using two methods. (1) Electron impact (EI-MS) and chemical ionization mass spectrometry: Electron impact mass spectra of the HPLC eluent fractions were measured with ionization at 70 eV in a Finnigan TSQ 700 (ion source temperature 150°C). Chemical ionization mass spectra were measured under the same conditions with NH_3 as reactant gas. The samples were introduced directly into the ion source and fractionally evaporized within the temperature range of 40–400°C; Under these EI-MS conditions thermic fragments in the higher mass range prevailed. (2) On-line HPLC-mass spectrometry: Unfractionated incubate solutions were measured on-line with HPLC-MS coupled with a thermospray interface. The equipment and the conditions were as follows. HPLC: 25 cm Hypersil C18, 5 µm, methanol : water 50 : 50, 0.1 *M* ammonium acetate, 1.6 ml/min, instrument Waters 600 MS. Thermospray: source temperature 220°C, vaporizer 96°C, electronic energy 100 V, repeller 9 V. MS: Finnigan TSQ 700, scan 70–500 daltons in 2 s.

Results

Biochemical Studies

Tissue Slices. The possible presence of metabolic transformation of Dexa was first studied in rat tissue slices. As documented by tables 1 and 2 Dexa is metabolized by renal and intestinal tissues in vitro, not however by testicular tissue. Liver slices exhibited only borderline activity. This parallels the pattern of B metabolism in rats (tables 1, 2) with the exception of testicular tissue, which in contrast to Dexa metabolized B quite actively. In general, metabolic activity of the slices for Dexa was only some 3–15% of that for B. Human kidney slices displayed a similar behavior when incubated with either Dexa or F (tables 1, 2). F has been used in this case since it is the physiological endogenous GCS in humans.

As shown in figure 1 is Dexa converted mainly into a more polar metabolite. This metabolite has tentatively been designated as 11-DH-Dexa on the ground of cochromatography experiments with an authentic metabolite. MS proof for the identity of the metabolite with 11-DH-Dexa is presented below. Consequently, the metabolic activity listed in tables 1 and 2 is designated 'oxidase activity'.

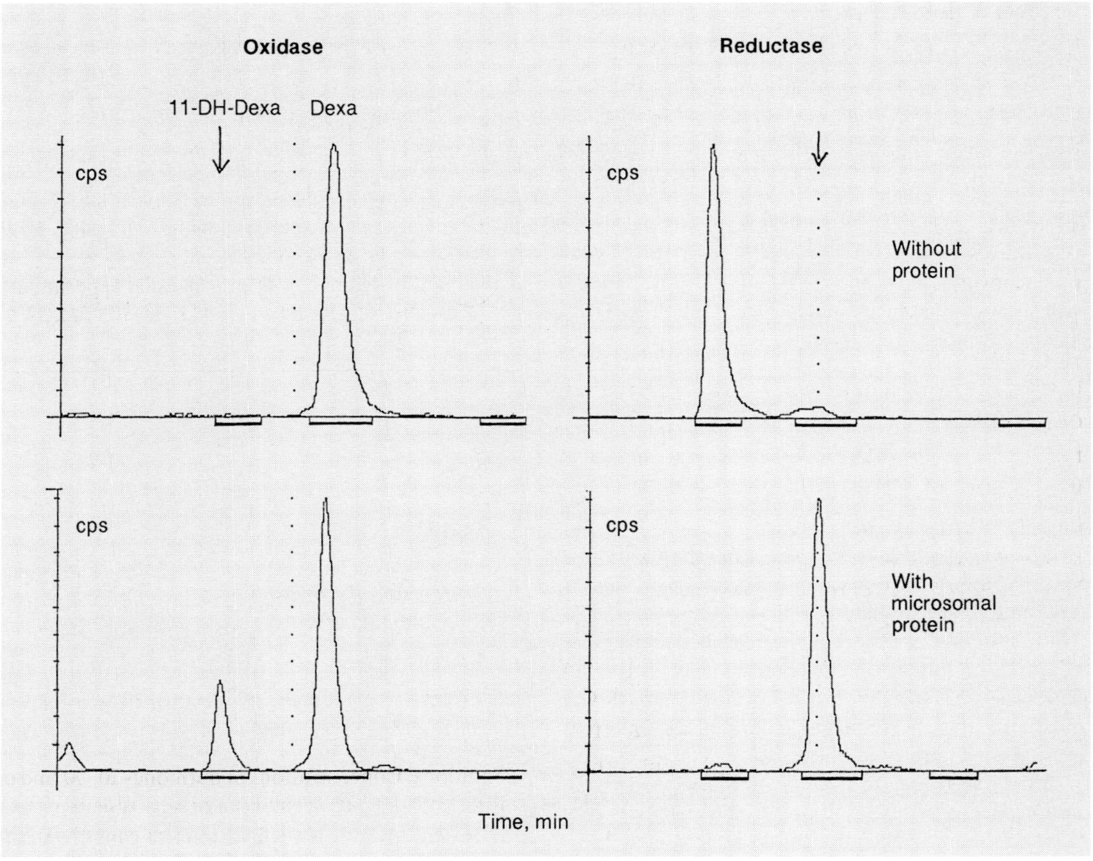

Fig. 1. Radiochromatograms of incubation of rat renal microsomes with Dexa (10^{-9} *M*, 200 μg protein) and 11-DH-Dexa (10^{-9} *M*, 750 μg protein), in 10 m*M* HEPES, pH 8.0, 37°C, 30 min.

In order to test the reverse reactions, designated as 'reductase activity', the equivalent 11-DH-metabolites were incubated. As shown in figure 1 11-DH-Dexa was exclusively converted to Dexa; the same holds true for 11-DH-B which was rapidly reduced to B by rat kidney slices, and for 11-DH-F which was converted to F by human renal tissue. It is pertinent to note that the apparent reductase activity for 11-DH-Dexa was higher than that for 11-DH-F and 11-DH-B, respectively. This is opposite to the oxidase pattern discussed above.

Homogenates. Homogenates of rat kidney and testicle were incubated in order to compare the apparent oxidase activity of 11β-HSD after cell disrupture with that of slices and to test the cosubstrate preference of the reaction (table 3). Again renal homogenate was more active in converting Dexa than testicular homogenate, the latter being devoid of activity even in the presence of added cosubstrates in high concentrations. Oxidase activity of kidney material displayed a clear preference for NAD^+ over $NADP^+$, both in the case of conversion of Dexa and of B. As in slices oxidation of Dexa was less effective than that of B. Oxidative activity for B in testicular homogenate was somewhat more effective in the presence of $NADP^+$. In order to study the cosubstrate preference under better-controlled conditions and to evaluate the effects of enzyme inhibition we turned to studies with microsomes.

Microsomal Fractions. With isolated microsomes we tested the metabolic activity of three organs, confirming essentially the previously observed differences in activity of kidney (high microscomal activity) and liver as well as testicles (borderline to zero activity) (fig. 1, fig. 2). It was also confirmed that the renal enzyme system is more sensitive to NAD^+ than to $NADP^+$ as cosubstrate. As in the slice studies microsome experiments were carried out in parallel with B. The data are presented in figure 2. In accordance with our previous observations all 3 microsomal fractions actively converted the endogenous GCS. Interestingly the renal microsomes reacted more actively in the presence of NAD^+, in contrast to hepatic and testicular microsomes which displayed higher activities with $NADP^+$.

Inhibition of Microsomal Dexa Degradation. Using rat renal microsomes we tested the effect of gly.ac. on the metabolism of Dexa and B. In both sets of experiments gly.ac. effectively inhibited conversion of Dexa as well as of B (fig. 3). The latter finding has already been published by us [15, 16]. Inhibition of steroid transformation by gly.ac. occurred in the presence of $NADP^+$ or NAD^+, respectively. Since gly.ac. predominantly inhibits 11-β-HSD [13–16] it can be concluded that Dexa undergoes oxidation at C_{11}.

Inhibition of Dexa degradation by rat renal microsomes could also be achieved by incubating microsomal fractions with Dexa (10^{-9} to 10^{-5} *M*) in the presence of B. This is not surprising since B, as demonstrated above, has a high affinity to the apparent CS degradation system. As documented by figure 4 Dexa degradation is completely inhibited in the presence of a 10^{-5} *M* B. Figure 4 demonstrates inhibition of Dexa degradation over the whole concentration range tested with NAD^+ and $NADP^+$, respectively. It is noteworthy that even at equimolar concentrations (10^{-5} *M*) B effectively inhibited degradation of Dexa.

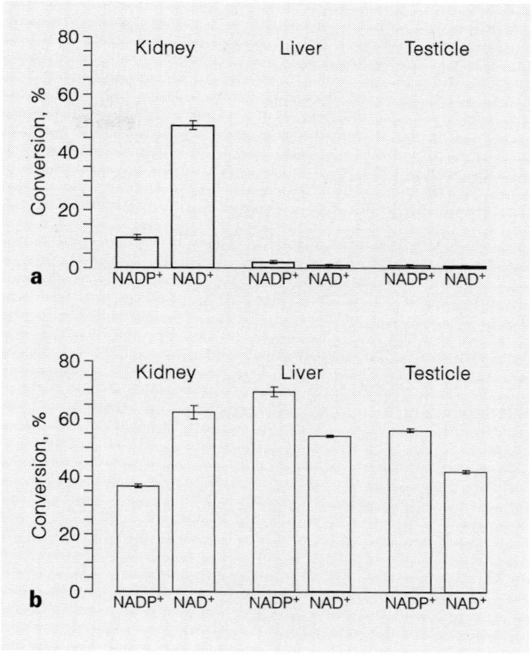

Fig. 2. Conversion of Dexa (**a**) and of B (**b**) by different microsomal fractions (note the difference in protein concentrations in the 2 sets of experiments). Conditions: Concentrations of hormones 10^{-9} *M* and of cosubstrates 10^{-3} *M*. Incubation of microsomal protein (200 μg for Dexa experiments and 10 μg for B experiments) in 10 m*M* HEPES, pH 8.0, 37 °C, 30 min.

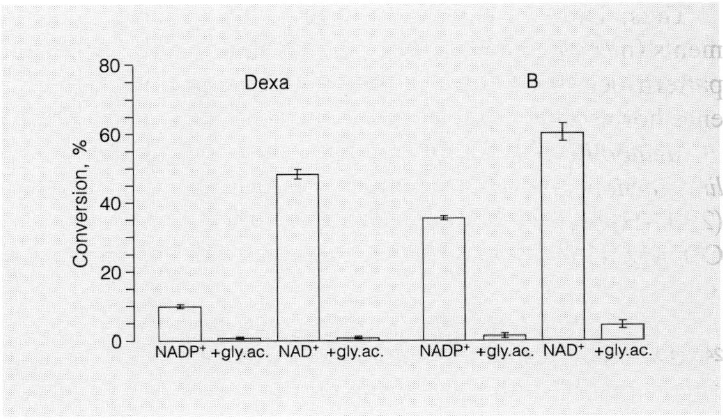

Fig. 3. Inhibition of Dexa degradation and B degradation by gly.ac. Conditions: Concentrations of hormones 10^{-9} *M*, of cosubstrates 10^{-3} *M* and of gly.ac. 10^{-7} *M*. Incubation of rat renal microsomal protein (200 μg for Dexa experiments and 10 μg for B experiments) in 10 m*M* HEPES, pH 8.0, 37 °C, 30 min.

Mass Spectrometry

EI-MS of the *Dexa fraction* revealed:

m/z 392 (2;M^+), 312 (20; M^+-HF-$COCH_2OH$-H), 294 (2;312-H_2O), 284 (4;312-CO);

242 (12; 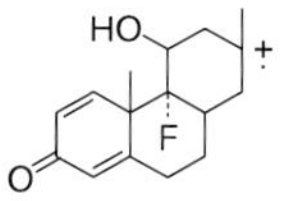 -HF),

122 (100; 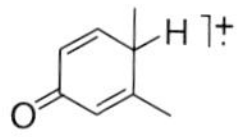),

121 (47; 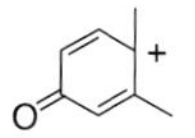).

HPLC-MS-coupling with thermospray interface of the *unseparated solution* at the position of *Dexa* revealed:

m/z 393 (100;$M+H^+$), 375 (17;393-H_2O), 363 (9;393-CH_2O), 333 (20;393-$COCH_2OH$-H).

This is equivalent to:

$C_{22}H_{29}FO_5$, MW:392

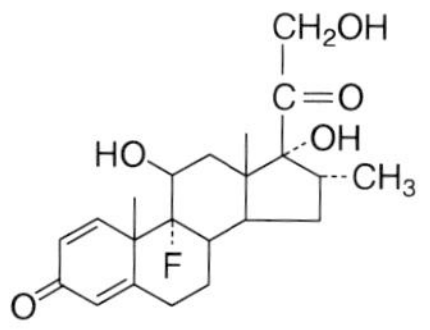

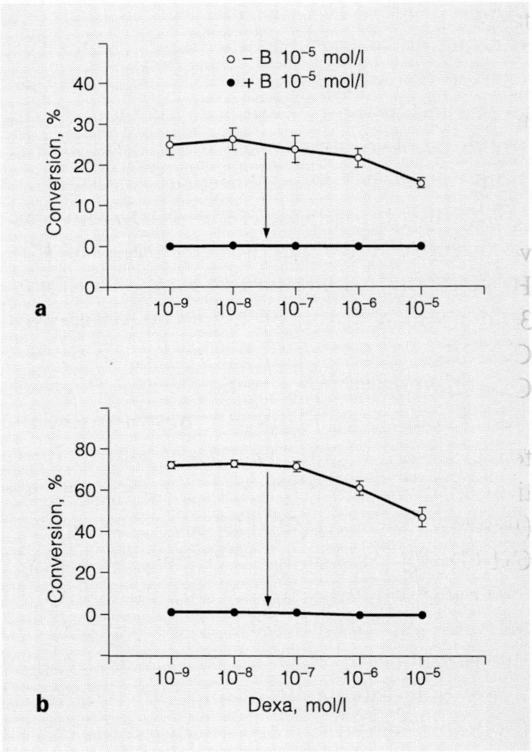

Fig. 4. Conversion of Dexa in different concentrations by rat renal microsomes with and without addition of 10^{-5} *M* B. Conditions: Incubation of 200 μg microsomal protein with 10^{-3} *M* $NADP^+$ (**a**) or NAD^+ (**b**) respectively, in 10 m*M* HEPES, pH 8.0, 37 °C, 30 min.

Thus, Dexa revealed the expected fragments (m/z values at 312, 242, 122, 121) and a pattern identical to that of the authentic reference hormone.

Metabolite of Dexa EI-MS of the *metabolite fraction* revealed: m/z 390 (3;M^+), 372 (2;M^+-H_2O), 360 (8;M^+-CH_2O), 330 (89;M^+-$COCH_2OH$-H), 310 (5;330-HF),

240 (18; 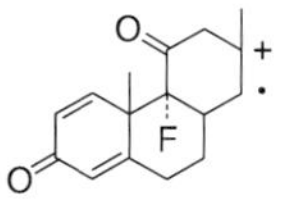 -HF),

239 (24; 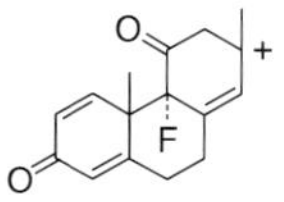 -HF),

122 (74; 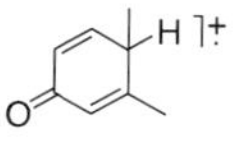),

121 (100; 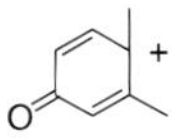).

CI/NH_3MS of the *metabolite fraction* revealed: m/z 408 (5;M+NH_4^+), 391 (28;M+H^+), 373 (12;391-H_2O), 361 (5;391-CH_2O), 348 (28;408-$COCH_2OH$-H), 331 (100;391-$COCH_2OH$-H), 313 (31;331-H_2O), 285 (2;313-CO).

HPLC-MS-coupling with thermospray interface of the *unseparated solution* at the position of the *metabolite peak* revealed: m/z 391 (100;M+H^+), 373 (20;391-H_2O), 361 (9;391-CH_2O), 331 (9;391-$COCH_2OH$-H).

This is equivalent to:

$C_{22}H_{27}FO_5$, MW:390

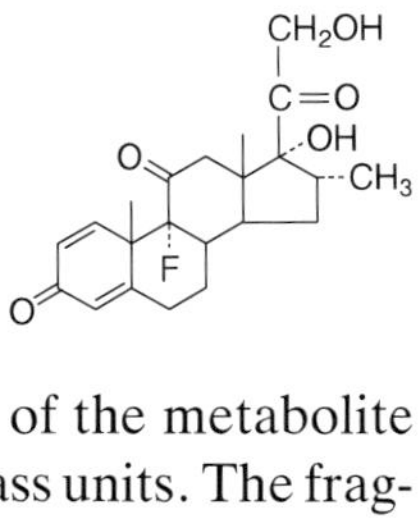

Thus, the molecular ion of the metabolite is smaller than Dexa by 2 mass units. The fragment pattern of the EI-MS with m/z 330, 240, 239, 122 and 121 prove that rings A, B and D as well as the side chain of the steroid skeleton are unchanged. Loss of 2 masses, therefore, must have occurred in ring C. This is compatible with conversion of the C-11 hydroxyl group into the respective C-11 keto group.

Discussion

The present study provides direct proof that the synthetic GCS dexamethasone is metabolized in several mammalian tissues by an enzyme system which reversibly oxidizes C_{11}-OH or reduces $C_{11}=O$ groups of the steroid skeleton. Particular activity could be demonstrated in CS target organs such as kidney and rectum. The main metabolite detected with our in vitro technique seemed to be 11-DH-Dexa. This assumption was first derived from the comparison of retention times of the respective metabolite with an authentic sample and from the fact that gly.ac. and B inhibited the production of the metabolite. Gly.ac. is a potent inhibitor of 11β-HSD [13–16]. B itself is a substrate for this enzyme system and competes with Dexa.

Metabolism of Dexa and other 9α-fluorinated CS has previously been studied under various physiological and clinical conditions. Bush et al. [5, 6, 32] working with homogenates and microsomes from rat + guinea pig livers tested the efficiency of the different 11-hydroxylated steroids as substrates for 11β-HSD. It was observed that CS with a halogen substitution in the 9α-position were protected from oxidation perhaps by steric prevention. The related 11-ketones in contrast underwent enhanced reduction. Our present results agree qualitatively with the notion that the 9α-fluorinated CS Dexa is less actively oxidized than for example B in rat preparations of F in human preparations. The more sensitive technique used here, however, permitted us to establish that in fact Dexa is to a significant extent oxidized at C_{11}. We also confirm the observation of Bush and Mahesh [5] and Bush et al. [6] that the reverse reaction, i.e. reduction of the $C_{11} = O$ group of Dexa, is enhanced as compared to that of 11-DH-B or 11-DH-F.

Several previous studies revealed different results regarding the metabolism of 9α-fluorinated CS, depending on species and biological system used. Hague et al. [18] observed that in man after intravenous administration Dexa is actively metabolized and that three unconjugated polar metabolites of unknown identity appear in the urine. More recently it has been reported that 6β-OH-Dexa is the main urinary metabolite in man [19]. In rats intraperitoneal injection of ^{3}H-Dexa led to the urinary excretion of unmetabolized Dexa as well as of a polar metabolite, likely to be 6β-OH-Dexa [20]. *Xenopus laevis*-derived A 6 cells in culture also convert Dexa into the 6β-OH metabolite [21]. In the urine of horses the main metabolite of injected Dexa was identified as 9αF-16α methyl-6β, 11β, 16β trihydroxy-1,4-androstadiene-3,17 dione [22]. Formation of 6-OH-Dexa in the rat was verified by English et al. [23] who in addition to unmetabolized Dexa detected 6-OH-Dexa and 20-dihydro-Dexa in rat urine after oral administration. The site of formation of the excreted metabolites was not defined. Oxidation at C_{11} in the whole organism has also been demonstrated for betamethasone by the demonstration of the 11-dehydro-metabolite in saliva and urine of man [7, 24]. Triamcinolone, another 9α-fluorinated corticoid, seems to be converted mainly into 6β-OH-triamcinolone [25, 26].

11β-HSD is a complex and heterogeneous enzyme system [27–31]. This is also indicated by the apparent cosubstrate preference of 11β-HSD in different tissues and under different conditions. Bush and Mahesh [5], Bush et al. [6] and Bush [32] observed only minimal activity of 11β-HSD with NAD^+ but a high activity with $NADP^+$. Koerner [33] and Koerner and Hellman [34], also found that $NADP^+$ was the more efficient cofactor in several tissues. The same was reported by Peterson et al. [35]. In contrast Hurlock and Talalay [36] observed roughly equal effectiveness of $NADP^+$ and NAD^+. In our studies cosubstrate preference of 11β-HSD was clearly heterogeneous. Apparent oxidase activity of 11β-HSD in rat and human kidney homogenate and microsomes was higher in the presence of NAD^+, regardless of the substrate hormone (Dexa, B or F). In 11β-HSD preparations from rat liver and testicle the $NADP^+$/H system was more effective. Striking was the preference of human liver homogenates for $NADP^+$ over NAD^+ by a factor of 10. This behavior altogether is another indication of the heterogeneity of the 11β-HSD system, perhaps for the presence of isoenzymes. This is in accordance with previous studies [37] and will be addressed in detail in a following paper.

The present finding of metabolic transformation of Dexa leading to 11-dehydro-Dexa is in congruence with recent observations which were obtained in rat rectal colon [38]. In stripped preparations in vitro aldosterone and Dexa elicited a stimulation of electrogenic Na^+ transport albeit with different potencies: K_M(n*M*) of 1.1 (aldosterone) and of 37, (Dexa). Maximum stimulation of Na^+ transport and apparent Hill kinetics for both steroids were not significantly different. However, when 11β-HSD of the rectal colon was blocked by gly.ac. (10^{-6} *M*) apparent mineralocorticosteroid (MCS) potency of Dexa increased: 10 n*M* Dexa exerted MCS action not different from that of 10 n*M* aldosterone. The MCS effect of Dexa could be inhibited by the new anti-MCS mespirenone® (courtesy of Schering). Since gly.ac. does not affect the MCS potency of aldosterone, this series of results documents that Dexa exerts MCS activity, which is intensified when metabolic degradation of the hormone at C_{11} is inhibited. It cannot, at present, conclusively be decided whether or not the MCS effect of inhibition of 11β-HSD exerted in the presence of Dexa favors increased binding of Dexa to MCS receptors, to GCS receptors or to both with subsequent stimulation of Na^+ transport.

Acknowledgement

This study has been supported by the Deutsche Forschungsgemeinschaft (Hi 97/16.1-6). Parts of it have been presented at the 7th European Colloquium on Renal Physiology. Napoli, June 13–16, 1992 [39].

References

1 Marver D: Evidence of corticosteroid action along the nephron. Am J Physiol 1984;246:F11–F123.
2 Träger L: Steroidhormone, Biosynthese, Stoffwechsel, Wirkung. Berlin, Springer, 1977.
3 Liddle GW: Tests of pituitary-adrenal suppressibility in the diagnosis of Cushing's syndrome. J Clin Endocrinol 1960;20:1539–1560.
4 Meikle AW, Tyler FH: Potency and duration of action of glucocorticoids. Effects of hydrocortisone, prednisone, and dexamethasone on human pituitary-adrenal function. Am Med 1977;63:200–207.
5 Bush IE, Mahesh VB: Metabolism of 11-oxygenated steroids. Biochem J 1964;93:236–255.
6 Bush IE, Hunter SA, Meigs RA: Metabolism of 11-oxygenated steroids. Metabolism in vitro by preparations of liver. Biochem J 1968;107:239–258.
7 Murphy D, West HF, Bethel AM: Some aspects of the metabolism and disposition of betamethasone. Acta Endocrinol 1964;45:498–508.
8 Dumasia MC, Horner MW, Houghton E, Moss MS: The urinary excretion and metabolism of dexamethasone in the horse. Biochem Soc Trans 1976;4:119–121.
9 Kobayashi N, Schulz W, Hierholzer K: Corticosteroid metabolism in rat kidney in vitro. IV. Subcellular sites of 11-hydroxy-steroid dehydrogenase activity. Pflügers Arch 1987;408:46–53.
10 Schulz W, Lichtenstein I, Siebe H, Hierholzer K: Isoelectric focusing analysis of detergent extracted renal 11β-hydroxysteroid dehydrogenase. J Steroid Biochem 1989;32:581–590.
11 Remmer H, Greim H, Schenkmann JB, Estabrook RW: Methods of the elevation of hepatic microsomal mixed function oxidase levels and cytochrome P-450; in Fleischer S, Estabrook RW (eds): Methods in Enzymology. New York, Academic Press, 1967, vol 10, pp 703–708.
12 Hübscher G, West GR: Specific assays of some phosphatase in subcellular fractions of small intestinal mucosa. Nature 1965;205:799–800.
13 Stewart PM, Valentino R, Wallace AM, Burt D, Shackleton CHL, Edwards CRW: Mineralocorticoid activity of liquorice: 11-β-Hydroxysteroid dehydrogenase deficiency comes of age. Lancet 1987;ii:821–823.
14 Monder C, Stewart PM, Lakshmi R, Valentino R, Burt D, Edwards CRW: Liquorice inhibits corticosteroid 11-β-dehydrogenase of rat kidney and liver: In vivo and in vitro studies. Endocrinology 1989;125:1046–1053.
15 Hierholzer K, Siebe H, Fromm M: Inhibition of 11β-hydroxysteroid dehydrogenase and its effect on epithelial sodium transport. Kidney Int 1990;38:673–678.
16 Bühler H, Kobayashi N, Lichtenstein I, Perschel FH, Siebe H, Hierholzer K: Reversible inhibition of renal 11β-hydroxysteroid dehydrogenase (11β-HSD) by steroids, structure-function relationship. Nieren Hochdruckkr 1990;19:374.
17 Schulz W, Kobayashi N, Siebe H, Hierholzer K: Studies on renal metabolism of corticosterone. Miner Electrolyte Metab 1987;13:355.
18 Hague N, Thrasher K, Werk EE, Knowles HC, Sholiton LJ: Studies on dexamethasone metabolism in man: Effect of diphenylhydantoin. J Clin Endocrinol Metab 1972;34:44–50.
19 Minagawa K, Kasuya Y, Baba S, Knapp G, Skelly JP: Identification and quantification of 6β-hydroxydexamenthasone as a major urinary metabolite of dexamethasone in man. Steroids 1986;47:175–188.
20 Rice MJ, Tredger M, Chakraborty J, Parke DV: The metabolism of dexamethasone in the rat. Biochem Soc Trans 1974;2:107–109.
21 Matsuzaki K, Miyazaki T, Yasuda K: Formation of 6 beta-hydroxydexamethasone from dexamethasone by A6 cells. Endocrinol Jpn 1991;38:131–135.
22 Skrabalak DS, Maylinn GA: Dexamethasone metabolism in the horse. Steroids 1982;39:233–244.
23 English J, Chakraborty J, Marks V: The metabolism of dexamethasone in the rat – Effect of phenytoin. J Steroid Biochem 1975;6:65–68.
24 Butler J, Gray CH: The metabolism of betamethasone. J Endocrinol 1970;46:379–390.

25 Florini JR, Smith LL; Buyske DA: Metabolic fate of a synthetic corticosteroid (triamcinolone) in the dog. J Biol Chem 1961;236:1038–1043.
26 Kripalani KJ, Cohen AI, Weliky I, Schreiber EC: Metabolism of triamcinolone acetonide-21-phosphate in does, monkeys, and rats. J Pharm Sci 1975;64:1351–1359.
27 Monder C, Shackleton CHL: 11β-Hydroxysteroid dehydrogenase: Fact or fancy? Steroids 1984;44: 383–417.
28 Kapturczak M, Bühler H, Lichtenstein I, Hierholzer K: Isoforms of 11β-hydroxysteroid dehydrogenase (11β-HSD) activity along the mouse nephron. Wissenschaftswoche im Klinikum Steglitz 1991; in Forschungsprojekte am Klinikum Steglitz, V.i.S.d.P.: Forschungskommission des Universitätsklinikums Steglitz, Hausdruckerei des UKS. 212–214. Submitted.
29 Bühler H, Perschel FH, Hierholzer K: Inhibition of rat 11-hydroxysteroid dehydrogenase by steroidal compounds and triterpenoids; structure-function relationship. BBA 1991;1075:206–212.
30 Hierholzer K, Bühler H, Perschel FH: Target Cell Metabolism of Corticosteroids Mediating Antisteroid Effects. 11th Int Congr Nephrol Symp Mol Actions Diuretics, Tokyo, 1990. Tokyo, Springer, 1991, pp 1122–1135.
31 Castello R, Schwarting R, Müller C, Hierholzer K, Lichtenstein I: Immunohistochemical localization of 11-hydroxysteroid dehydrogenase in rat kidney with a monoclonal antibody. Renal Physiol Biochem 1989;12:320–327.
32 Bush IE: 11β-Hydroxysteroid dehydrogenase: Contrast between studies in vivo and studies in vitro. Adv Biosci 1969;3:23–40.
33 Koerner DR: 11β-Hydroxysteroid dehydrogenase of lung and testis. Endocrinology 1966;79:935–938.
34 Koerner DR, Hellmann L: Effect of thyroxine administration on the 11-β-hydroxysteroid dehydrogenase in rat liver and kidney. Endocrinology 1964;75:592–601.
35 Petersen NA, Chaikoff IL, Jones C: The in vitro conversion of cortisol to cortisone by subcellular brain fractions of young and adult rats. Neurochemistry 1965;12:273–278.
36 Hurlock B, Talalay P: Microsomal 3α- and 11β-hydroxysteroid dehydrogenases. Arch Biochem Biophys 1959;80:468–470.
37 Hierholzer K, Perschel FH, Bühler H, Fromm M: Target organ metabolism of corticosteroids: Studies on 11β-hydroxysteroid dehydrogenase; in Bonvalet JP, Farman N, Lombès M, Rafestin-Oblin ME (eds): Aldosterone Fundamental Aspects. Colloques Inserm. Paris, Libbey Eurotext, 1991, vol 215, pp 97–107.
38 Fromm M, Epple HJ, Schulzke JD, Hierholzer K: Dose-response of aldosterone and ten other corticosteroids on electrogenic Na^+ transport in rat rectal colon in vitro; in Bonvalet JP, Farman N, Lombès M, Rafestin-Oblin ME (eds): Aldosterone Fundamental Aspects. Colloques Inserm. Paris, Libbey Eurotext, 1991, vol 215, p 334.
39 Siebe H, Wang D, Bühler H, Lichtenstein I, Hierholzer K: Dexamethasone in metabolized by rat renal microsomes. 7th European Colloquium on Renal Physiology, Naples, Castel dell'Ovo, June 13–16, 1992. Renal Physiol Biochem 1992;210:179.

Renal Physiol Biochem 1993;16:89–92

Carla Zoja[a]
Alessandro Rambaldi[a]
Giuseppe Remuzzi[a,b]

[a] Mario Negri Institute for Pharmacological Research, and
[b] Division of Nephrology and Dialysis, Ospedali Riuniti di Bergamo, Bergamo Italy

Interleukin-1 and Glomerular Mesangial Cells

Key Words
Mesangial cells
Interleukin-1 gene
Interleukin-1 receptor
Interleukin-1 receptor antagonist
Interleukin-6 gene
Interleukin-8 gene

Abstract

Our previous in vitro study demonstrated that interleukin-1 (IL-1) stimulates gene expression and production of leukocyte chemotactic factors, colony-stimulating factors and interleukin-6 in human mesangial cells in culture. Here we investigated whether IL-1 regulates its own gene expression in human mesangial cells. Northern blot experiments showed that IL-1 induced IL-1 mRNA expression in a dose-dependent manner. The action of IL-1 on mesangial cells was mediated through the IL-1 receptor type I, which is constitutively expressed by mesangial cells. Recombinant IL-1 receptor antagonist blocked the IL-1 mRNA as well as interleukin-6 and interleukin-8 gene expression induced by IL-1. These data support the crucial role played by IL-1 in regulating mesangial cell cytokine genes within the glomerulus during immunological or inflammatory processes.

Background

Interleukin-1 (IL-1) represents a family of proteins that have a central function in inflammatory and immunologic processes by affecting various organs and tissues [1, 2]. In recent years evidence has emerged to indicate the potential role of IL-1 derived from both intrinsic mesangial cells and/or macrophages infiltrating glomeruli as mediator of glomerular inflammation and disease progression. Lovett et al. [3, 4] and Lovett and Larsen [5] reported that Il-1 is expressed and secreted by cultured mesangial cells and that it promotes mesangial cell proliferation. Moreover, the same authors documented the capability of IL-1 to stimulate mesangial cell synthesis of inflammatory prostanoids [6]. Findings that IL-1 stimulates an increase of mRNAs coding for type I and IV collagen and fibronectin in rat mesangial cells [7] and that gene expression of IL-1 is increased in kidneys of rats with im-

Dr. Giuseppe Remuzzi
Mario Negri Institute for Pharmacological Research
Via Gavazzeni, 11
I-24125 Bergamo (Italy)

1011–6524/93/0162–0089 $2.75/0

mune complex glomerulonephritis [8] are also of support to the role of IL-1 as mediator of glomerular injury.

We have recently shown that IL-1 stimulates gene expression of interleukin-6, leukocyte chemotactic factors interleukin-8 and monocyte chemotactic protein-1, and colony-stimulating factors in cultured human mesangial cells. Cytokine gene expression was accompanied by active secretion of corresponding peptides in mesangial cell supernatant [9].

Here we wanted to determine whether IL-1 induces its own gene expression in human glomerular mesangial cells and whether the action of IL-1 on mesangial cells is mediated through the IL-1 receptor type I.

Methods

Culture of Mesangial Cells

Mesangial cells were obtained from collagenase-treated isolated human glomeruli and cultured in RPMI 1640 medium supplemented with 15 m*M* N-2-hydroxyethylpiperazine-N′-2-ethanesulfonic acid (HEPES, Sigma Chemical Co., St. Louis, Mo.), 0.6 U/ml of insulin (Actrapid HM, Novo Industri A/S, Copenhagen, Denmark), 2 m*M* glutamine (Gibco Laboratories, Grand Island, N.Y.), 0.1 m*M* nonessential amino acids (Sigma), 1 m*M* sodium pyruvate (Gibco), 100 U/ml of penicillin, 100 μg/ml streptomycin, 250 ng/ml of fungizone and 17% fetal calf serum (Hyclone, Logan, Utah) as previously described [9]. Confluent cells were passed by being washed with Ca^{2+}-free Mg^{2+}-free Hanks' balanced solution followed by incubation with 0.025% trypsin-0.5 m*M* EDTA and resuspension in complete RPMI 1640 medium. Cells were used between passages 5 and 10. They were identified, and their purity was assessed by phase contrast and electron microscopy and by staining for intermediate filaments and surface antigens by the avidin-biotin immunoperoxidase method as previously described [9].

Incubation of Mesangial Cells

Confluent human mesangial cells grown in 100-mm plastic dishes were incubated for 6 h at 37 °C in 5 ml of RPMI 1640 medium with 10% fetal calf serum in the absence or presence of human recombinant IL-1β (10 ng/ml; provided by Dr. D. Boraschi, Sclavo, Siena, Italy; SA of 10^7 U/mg of protein), containing less than 0.3 pg of endotoxin/μg by the Limulus amebocyte lysate assay. When dose-response studies were performed, mesangial cells were incubated for 6 h with 1, 10, and 100 ng/ml of IL-1β. In selected experiments, mesangial cells were also incubated with human recombinant tumor necrosis factor-α (TNF-α; 10 ng/ml; Cetus, Emeryville, Calif.; SA of 10^7 U/mg of protein), bacterial lipopolysaccharide (LPS, 1 μg/ml; *Escherichia coli* 0111:B4, Difco Laboratories, Detroit, Mich.), transforming growth-factor-β (TGF-β, 10 ng/ml; provided by Dr. M. Palladino, Genentech, San Francisco, Calif.) and human recombinant interleukin-6 (IL-6, 100 U/ml; provided by Dr. S. Gillis, Immunex, Seattle, Wash.). In some experiments before the addition of IL-1β, mesangial cells were pretreated for 15 min with human recombinant IL-1 receptor antagonist (IL-1ra) (100 and 1,000 ng/ml; provided by Dr. R. C. Thompson, Synergen, Boulder, Colo.). At the end of the incubation, the cells were used for total cellular RNA preparation by guanidium isothiocyanate/cesium chloride ultracentrifugation.

Northern Blot Analysis

Northern blot experiments were performed as previously described [9]. IL-1β cDNA probe was kindly provided by Dr. S. Clark (Genetics Institute, Cambridge, Mass.). A human IL-1 receptor (IL-1R) cDNA (HindIII-EcoRI fragment of 477 base pairs) [10] was obtained through the courtesy of Dr. S. K. Dower (Immunex, Seattle, Wash.). MDNCF/IL-8 cDNA probe was kindly provided by Dr. K. Matsushima (Laboratory of Molecular Immunoregulation, National Cancer Institute, Bethesda, Md.) [11]. IL-6 mRNA was detected by the use of the BanII-BanII fragment (620 base pairs) of the human IL-6 cDNA (generously provided by Dr. G. Wong and Dr. S. Clark, Genetics Institute).

Results and Comments

Northern blot experiments have demonstrated that IL-1β (1–100 ng/ml) induces a dose-dependent increase of IL-1β mRNA levels with respect to unstimulated mesangial cells. Thus in mesangial cells, as it occurs in monocytes and endothelial cells, IL-1 acts as a stimulus of its own gene expression. Since cells participating in the process of glomerular inflammation, namely macrophages, blood monocytes and neutrophils, and endothelial cells are sources of IL-1, the pathway by which IL-1 upregulates its own gene expression in mesangial cells might be an important process of glomerular damage.

Two structurally distinct receptors for IL-1 have been identified with differential cellular distribution [12, 13]. The IL-1R type I of 80 kD is expressed on T cells, fibroblasts and endothelial cells [10, 14], whereas the IL-1R type II of 68 kD has been found on B-cells and on myelomonocytic cells [15–17]. We took advantage of the recent purification and cloning of the IL-1R type I [10, 14] to assess whether mesangial cells express the IL-1R gene and to clarify how IL-1R gene expression is regulated. We have found that human mesangial cells in culture constitutively express the 80-kD IL-1R type I. No modulation of the IL-1R mRNA was observed when mesangial cells were exposed to IL-1β, TNF-α, LPS, TGF-β or IL-6.

With additional experiments we have shown that treatment of mesangial cells with recombinant IL-1ra at the concentration of 100 ng/ml resulted in a partial inhibition of IL-1β-induced mRNA expression. When the concentration of 1,000 ng/ml was used it was capable of completely suppressing the IL-1β transcript.

It is of interest that IL-1ra also blocked mesangial cell IL-6 and IL-8 gene expression induced by IL-1. Since IL-6 and IL-8 are both implicated in inflammatory or immunologic processes occurring at glomerular levels [18, 19] one can speculate that inhibiting these cytokines may indeed reduce the glomerular damage. Altogether these data support the crucial role of IL-1 in regulating mesangial cell cytokine genes and might indicate the existence of an IL-1-mediated positive feedback loop controlling the secretion of active cytokines within the glomerulus when an immunologic or inflammatory injury takes place.

It is possible to speculate that the antagonism of IL-1 binding to the IL-1R might block secondary responses triggered by an immunologic insult to the kidney. Thus, if this operates in vivo, the use of IL-1ra as a therapeutic agent for glomerulonephritis might represent an exciting possibility in future years.

References

1 Dinarello CA: Biology of interleukin-1. FASEB J 1988;2:108–115.
2 Dinarello CA: Interleukin-1 and interleukin-1 antagonism. Blood 1991;77:1627–1652.
3 Lovett DH, Szamel M, Ryan JL, Sterzel RB, Gemsa D, Resch K: Interleukin 1 and the glomerular mesangium. I. Purification and characterization of a mesangial cell-derived autogrowth factor. J Immunol 1986;136:3700–3705.
4 Lovett DH, Ryan JL, Sterzel RB: Stimulation of rat mesangial cell proliferation by macrophage interleukin 1. J Immunol 1987;131:2473–2480.
5 Lovett DH, Larsen A: Cell cycle-dependent interleukin 1 gene expression by cultured glomerular mesangial cells. J Clin Invest 1988; 82:115–122.
6 Lovett DH, Resch K, Gemsa D: Interleukin 1 and the glomerular mesangium. II. Monokine stimulation of mesangial cell prostanoid secretion. Am J Pathol 1987;129:543–551.
7 Suzuki S, Ebihara I, Nakamura T, Tomino Y, Koide H: Effects of peptide growth factors on regulation of extracellular matrix gene expression in cultured rat mesangial cells (abstract). JASN 1991;2:446.
8 Werber HI, Emancipator SN, Tykocinski ML, Sedor JR: The interleukin 1 gene is expressed by rat glomerular mesangial cells and is augmented in immune complex glomerulonephritis. J Immunol 1987; 138:3207–3212.

9 Zoja C, Wang JM, Bettoni S, Sironi M, Renzi D, Chiaffarino F, Abboud HE, Van Damme J, Mantovani A, Remuzzi G, Rambaldi A: Interleukin-1β and tumor necrosis factor-α induce gene expression and production of leukocyte chemotactic factors, colony-stimulating factors, and interleukin-6 in human mesangial cells. Am J Pathol 1991;138: 991–1003.

10 Sims JE, Acres RB, Grubin CE, McMahan CJ, Wignall JM, March CJ, Dower SK: Cloning the interleukin 1 receptor from human T cells. Proc Natl Acad Sci USA 1989; 86:8946–8950.

11 Matsushima K, Morishita K, Yoshimura T, Lavu S, Kobayashi Y, Lew W, Appella E, Kung HF, Leonard EJ, Oppenheim JJ: Molecular cloning of a human monocyte-derived neutrophil chemotactic factor (MDNCF) and the induction of MDNCF mRNA by interleukin 1 and tumor necrosis factor. J Exp Med 1988;167:1883–1893.

12 Bomsztyc K, Sims JE, Stanton TH, Slack J, McMahan CJ, Valentine MA, Dower SK: Evidence for different interleukin 1 receptors in murine B- and T-cell lines. Proc. Natl Acad Sci USA 1989;86:8034–8038.

13 Chizzonite R, Truitt T, Kilian PL, Stern AS, Nunes P, Parker KP, Kaffka KL, Chua AO, Lugg DK, Gubler U: Two high-affinity interleukin 1 receptors represent separate gene products. Proc Natl Acad Sci USA 1989;86:8029–8033.

14 Sims JE, March CJ, Cosmos D, Widmer MB, Mac Donald HR, McMahan CJ, Grubin CE, Wignall JM, Jackson JL, Call SM, Gillis S, Dower SK: cDNA expression cloning of the IL-1 receptor, a member of the immunoglobulin superfamily. Science 1988;241:585–589.

15 Matsushima K, Akahoshi T, Yamada M, Furutani Y, Oppenheim JJ: Properties of a specific interleukin-1 receptor on human Epstein-Barr virus-transformed B lymphocytes: Identity of the receptor for IL-α and IL-β. J Immunol 1986;136: 4496–4502.

16 Horuk R, Huang JJ, Covington M, Newton RC: A biochemical and kinetic analysis of the interleukin-1 receptor. Evidence for differences in molecular properties of IL-1 receptors. J Biol Chem 1987;262: 16275–16278.

17 Horuk R, McCubrey JA: The interleukin-1 receptor in Raji human B lymphoma cells. Biochem J 1989; 260:657–663.

18 Horii Y, Maraguchi A, Iwano M, Matsuda T, Hirayama T, Yamada H, Fujii Y, Dohi K, Ishikawa H, Ohmoto Y, Yoshizaki K, Hirano T, Kishimoto T: Involvement of IL-6 in mesangial proliferative glomerulonephritis. J Immunol 1989;143: 3949–3955.

19 Badr KF, Munger KA, Miller E: Increased glomerular synthesis of a novel monocyte-derived peptide agonist, neutrophil activating factor (NAF), during late nephrotoxic serum nephritis (NTS) in rats (abstract) Kidney Int 1990;37:362.

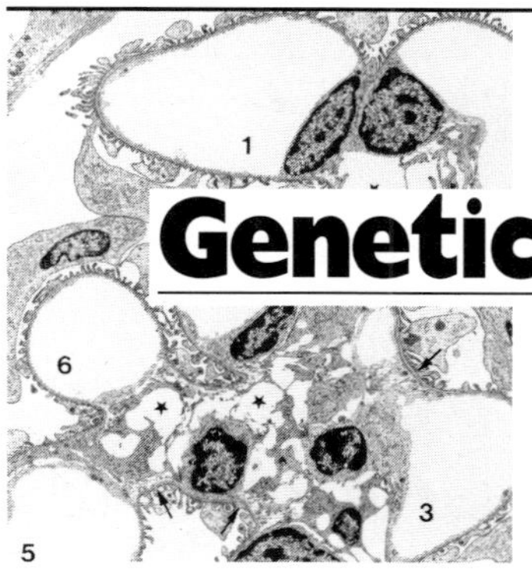

Experimental and Genetic Rat Models of Chronic Renal Failure

Editors: N. Gretz, M. Strauch

Animal models of chronic renal failure are useful research tools only when the selected model lends itself to providing the answer to a particular question. This practical book presents a broad spectrum of experimental and genetic rat models of chronic renal failure in such a way that their advantages, disadvantages and special features are clearly indicated. The information provided enables researchers to choose the appropriate model. This is especially important in the testing of therapeutic modalities. The book not only describes the induction and progression of renal failure, but also discusses factors, intrinsic to each model, which could considerably influence results. In addition, problems in the measurement of blood pressure and glomerular filtration rate are considered in detail.

This volume is an indispensable aid to all scientists working with animal models of renal failure, and is especially helpful to young researchers wishing to start with animal experiments.

Contents

Fields of Interest

Nephrology; Pharmacology; Biochemistry, Genetics, Hematology, Metabolism, Pathology, Physiology, Urology

Experimental and Genetic Rat Models of Chronic Renal Failure
Editors: Gretz, N.; Strauch, M. (Mannheim)
X + 344 p., 74 fig., 40 tab., hard cover, 1993
SFr. 248.– / DM 297.– / US$ 198.50
Prices subject to change
DM price for FRG, US$ price for USA only
ISBN 3–8055–5499–0

KI 93512

KARGER

Contributions to Nephrology (ISSN 0302–5144), **Vol. 101**
Series Editors: G.M. Berlyne, Brooklyn, N.Y.; S. Giovannetti, Pisa

Kidney, Proteins and Drugs: An Update

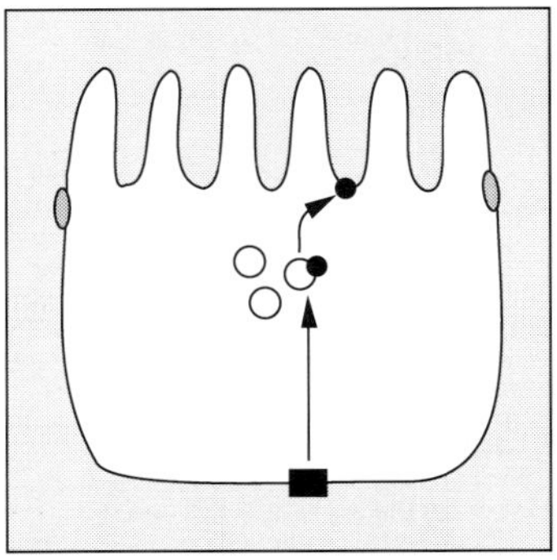

Editors:
Claudio Bianchi, Velio Bocci, Frank A. Carone, Ralph Rabkin

Facilitates more accurate diagnosis and therapy

The kidney plays a crucial role in the metabolism of many low molecular weight proteins. Many drugs and chemicals can injure the kidney and cause an increase in urinary proteins and enzymes. This publication reports the latest findings from experimental and clinical medicine on the renal handling of proteins and the nephrotoxicity of drugs and contrast media. Other areas of interest include renal physiology and pathophysiology, proteinuria, and the importance of urinary proteins and enzymes in the detection of kidney damage.

Updating the information presented in volume 83 of *Contributions to Nephrology*, this book is important reading for scientists and clinicians interested in the renal handling of proteins and the effects of drugs on the kidney.

Main Headings

Physiology and Pathophysiology
Renal Handling of Proteins
Proteinuria
Urinary Proteins and Enzymes to Detect Kidney Damage
Renal Handling and Nephrotoxicity of Drugs and Contrast Media

Fields of Interest

Nephrology;
Pharmacology;
Physiology;
Biochemistry,
Metabolism,
Urology

Contributions to Nephrology, Vol. 101
Kidney, Proteins and Drugs: An Update
7th International Symposium of Nephrology at Montecatini,
Montecatini Terme, October 1991
Editors: Bianchi, C. (Pisa); Bocci, V. (Siena); Carone, F.A. (Chicago, Ill.);
Rabkin, R. (Palo Alto, Calif.)
X + 270 p., 84 fig., 36 tab., hard cover, 1993
SFr. 248.– / DM 297.– / US$ 198.50
Prices subject to change · DM price for FRG, US$ price for USA only
Distributed in Japan exclusively by Igaku Shoin Ltd., Tokyo ISBN 3–8055–5668–3

KI 92767

KARGER